Triathlon
made easy

Zoë McDonald & Lisa Buckingham

in association with

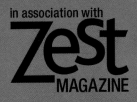

ZeSt
MAGAZINE

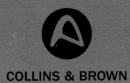

COLLINS & BROWN

First published in Great Britain in 2008
by Collins and Brown
10 Southcombe Street
London W14 0RA

An imprint of Anova Books

Distributed in the United States and Canada by
Sterling Publishing Co, 387 Park Avenue South,
New York, NY 10016, USA

Zest is the registered trademark of The Nationa
Magazine Company Ltd.

The authors have made every reasonable effort
contact all copyright holders. Any errors that ma
have occurred are inadvertent and anyone who t
any reason has not been contacted is invited to
write to the publishers so that a full
acknowledgement may be made in subsequent
editions of this work.

British Library Cataloguing in Publication Data.
A catalogue record for this title is available from
the British Library.

ISBN 9781843404330

Picture Credits: Triathlon event photos courtesy of
SportCam and Action Photo (page 4 and 5)
Illustrator Maxim Savva
Stylists Marianne de Vries, Kelly Moseley
Still-life photographer Derek Lomas
Cover photographer Neil Cooper

Repro by Spectrum Colour Ltd, UK
Printed in Times Offset (M) Sdn. Bhd, Malaysia

The exercise programmes in this
book are intended for people in
good health – if you have a
medical condition or are pregnant,
or have any other health concerns,
always consult your doctor before
starting out.

contents

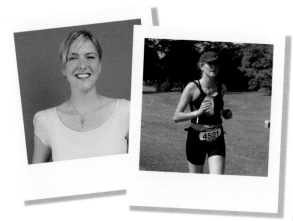

Zoë McDonald, 29, is a health and fitness journalist with 8 years' experience. She is *Zest*'s features editor

My fitness CV: Sports were not my strong point at school. I detested PE and was the slowest swimmer in my club. I even failed my cycling proficiency test. At uni, occasional swimming sessions to burn off my wine intake were my only attempt at exercise.

When I moved back to London after university, a sedentary magazine desk job got me thinking about exercise again. I began with a 20-minute running loop from my house, and signed up for my first race (a 5K) after a few months. The atmosphere was inspiring, and I vowed to keep it up. But numerous gym memberships started and lapsed, and my trainers gathered dust. Then I joined *Zest* magazine. Within months I was running regularly and I'd signed up for more 5K and 10Ks. Next came the Flora London Marathon – an incredible experience, but once I'd done it I needed a new challenge. Several girlfriends signed up for triathalons

and reported back that the races were great fun. I decided it was about time I overcame my fear of cycling, so signed up for my first race.

Worst moment: Building my cycling confidence was tough. I started commuting by bike, and found it nervewracking at first, but the benefits soon became clear. For my first triathlon (the Stratford 220), it bucketed with rain, which made the bike ride a little hairy, and my first open-water swim at the Mazda Blenheim Triathlon was a challenge (I wish I'd practised swimming in open water beforehand!).

Proudest moment: Completing my first triathlon – it felt like an impossible dream at first, but crossing the finish line was an unbeatable feeling, and despite nerves, torrential rain and a wobbly bike ride, I loved it! As this book goes to press, I'm training for my first Olympic-distance race (the Michelob Ultra London Triathlon).

Motivation secret: There's nothing quite as motivating as conditioning your body to be strong enough to swim, bike and run your way through a race with confidence, and training is a great stress-buster. If ever I feel like missing a session, I remind myself of how serene I'll feel afterwards!

Ultimate goal: To get faster on my bike and record a decent time in my first Olympic-distance race.

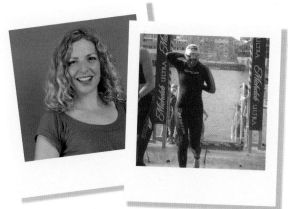

Lisa Buckingham, 29, is deputy health editor on *Best* magazine and contributing editor on *Zest*

Fitness CV: My love of sport has come with age. School athletics were always a bore and my attempts to play hockey at university petered out when I found that bar sports were my talent! That, combined with beer and a love of tuna-mayonnaise toasties, meant I left uni weighing 11st (I'm 5ft 6in).

After uni, I discovered adventure sports, learning to snowboard, surf, scuba-dive and rock-climb, and found to my surprise that I relished the thrill of new challenges.

In 2003 I was away surfing with a group of friends when I overheard two of the boys talking about sprint triathlons. I thought the distance sounded quite achievable (400m–750m swim, 20K bike and 5K run) and that's where it started. I did my first sprint tri that summer with a borrowed bike and no idea what I was doing, and have since done nine more. It's changed my body (I'm now 2st lighter) and I love the training, as I can do it all outside – I go for early morning swims in my local lido, ride my bike to work and run around a beautiful park. And the races are exhilarating – there's something hugely satisfying about knowing you've put three different sports together successfully.

Worst moment: The time I was so busy eating a Snickers bar and waving to my supporters at the beginning of the bike leg during my third triathlon that I crashed into the bollards and nearly took out one of the marshals...

Proudest moment: Crossing the finish line at the Michelob Ultra London Triathlon. It was my first Olympic-distance race and I was so astonished that I'd actually completed it. I was shaking with elation and couldn't stop grinning! I'd been really nervous about the length of the swim and whether I'd even finish in the August heat, but it all came together and I finished in 3:10.

My motivation secret: Signing up for races! Nothing will get me out of bed in the morning to train like the thought of not being able to finish on the day!

Ultimate goal: I've done sprint distance, I've done Olympic distance, now it's got be a half-Ironman (1.9K swim, 80K bike and 20K run). Be warned this is what happens when you get bitten by the triathlon bug!

Wondering if triathlon is for you? Perhaps you're tempted to get involved but have a list of doubts you'd like to settle first. Here, we outline the tri basics, present the answers to the commonest beginner's questions and concerns, and introduce you to four incredible people who transformed their bodies with triathlon...

1

why tri?

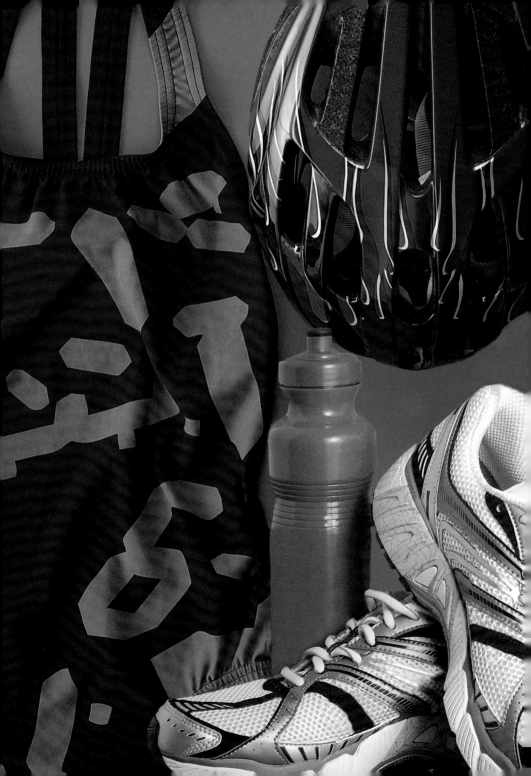

Anyone can tri

Yes, that means you! Whether you're a fit beginner looking for a new challenge or a complete novice searching for a motivating way to shape up, triathlon training (swimming, cycling and running) is the answer.

Triathlon is varied, delivers top-to-toe body benefits in a way no single sport could, and is far less likely to cause you an injury than any single-discipline training. If you're the competitive sort, it'll encourage you to stretch your mind and body in truly holistic style – being a triathlete means you get to be 360° fit!

Will it work for me?

If you approach the training in the right way, that is, not trying to do too much too quickly, or overdo one aspect of the training while neglecting the others, you'll soon see the benefits of triathlon training. It doesn't have to take many hours out of your week (a common triathlon myth), and you don't have to practise all three sports every time you train.

Triathlon training will transform your body, and can also deliver a life-changing mood and mindset makeover – we know, we've felt it! If you go about it the right way, your training time should become a real pleasure, the kind of 'me' time that leaves you feeling energised, confident and ready to face anything life can throw at you. So, if you're keen to get started, you're in the right place! *Triathlon Made Easy* has been designed to suit anyone –

from the self-confessed couch potato, to fit and fabulous gym bunnies who spin at lunchtime, love to run (and have the medals to prove it) and know their kick-buoy from their paddle in the pool.

We consulted expert coaches and triathletes, who helped us to create brilliant training sessions and three fabulous programmes – to suit every ability level. There will be a plan to suit you, whatever your fitness.

If you've got lingering concerns such as: 'I love to run and cycle, but hate swimming', 'I don't fancy the prospect of a soggy cycle', 'I don't want to spend a fortune on kit', or 'I don't have time', we've got the answers to reassure you.

No matter what your goal, *Triathlon Made Easy* will help to make your journey there fun, fresh and fascinating. Get ready to get hooked!

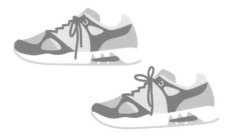

Need to know

The word 'triathlon' is ancient Greek in origin and refers to an event made up of three contests. But despite the archaic name, triathlon as we know it is a very new sport, which didn't get going until the 1970s in the USA, and didn't become an Olympic sport until the year 2000.

The majority of triathlons place swimming, cycling and running back to back, in that order, and your official finish time includes the 'transition' time you take switching kit and equipment between each leg of the race.

The official triathlon season in the UK runs from May to October. When it comes to racing distances, there are plenty to choose from. Below is a guide to the distances involved in each race. The races highlighted in bold are the ones we've focused on for our training plans for you.

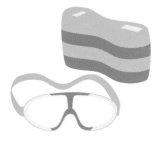

Event	Swim	Bicycle	Run
Super-Sprint or 'fun'	400m/0.25miles	10km/6.2miles	2.5km/1.5miles
Sprint	400–750m/ 0.25–0.5miles	20K/12.4miles	5K/3miles
Olympic	1500m/1mile	40K/24.8miles	10K/6.2miles
ITU-Long distance	3000m/2miles	80K/50miles	20K/12.4miles
Half-Ironman	1900m/1.2miles	90K/56miles	21.09K/ 13.1miles
Triathlon one 0 one (new)	3000m/2miles	130K/80.6miles	30K/18.6miles
Ironman	3800m/2.4miles	180K/112 miles	42.195K/ 26.2miles

10 reasons to tri

From cutting your risk of heart disease to building healthy bones, boosting your strength and transforming your shape, there are plenty of reasons your body will thank you for tri-ing.

1 You'll benefit your heart One person dies every 2 minutes in the UK as a result of coronary heart disease. Regular cardiovascular exercise (such as triathlon training) will cut your risk of developing heart disease in half.

2 You'll increase your chances of living longer Research at Harvard University in the USA found that people who burnt 2000 calories extra per week through exercise lived, on average, one to two years longer than people who burnt only 500 extra per week. On the Super-Sprint plan, you'll burn on average an extra 1300 calories per week and during an Olympic-distance race you may burn off more than 1900 calories!

3 It can help you to manage your weight Regular training will burn calories and increase your metabolism. Plus, the variety of tri training will help to keep you motivated for long-term healthy weight management.

4 You're less likely to get injured Triathlon training is good news for your body, particularly if you have sustained sports injuries in the past and you're worried about doing so again. An endurance runner is twice as likely to get injured as a triathlete. The reason is simple: muscles take 48 hours to recover after a training session, and triathletes train different muscles on different days, so the body has more of a chance to repair itself than if you're doing one type of exercise alone.

5 It's a great stress-buster Swimming, cycling and running qualify as what experts call 'moving meditation' thanks to their repetitive, rhythmic nature. This makes triathlon training more likely to deliver stress-relief benefits than, for example, squash or football. Triathlon training will reduce the levels of the stress hormone cortisol in your blood, enabling you to feel calmer, happier and more in control, with the benefits lasting long after your training finishes.

6 It'll improve your mood In a recent study, patients with depression who followed an exercise programme that included cycling and jogging for just three 30-minute sessions per week eliminated their symptoms within three months. Researchers at Duke

★ ★ ★ ★ ★ ★ ★ ★ ★ ★

University in the USA found that cross-training was as effective as a leading antidepressant at alleviating symptoms, and even more effective than the drugs at preventing the symptoms from returning in the future.

7 You'll get fit, fast! Even if you are unfit now, you'll be amazed at how quickly your strength, stamina and cardiovascular fitness builds with triathlon training. Although it is a challenge, it's more sensible to choose triathlon training to get fit than an individual sport. For a person who has done no exercise in recent years, starting to run five times a week is more likely to cause aches, pains and injury than doing, for example, two swims, two runs and a bike ride.

8 You'll build upper-body strength Running or cycling alone don't have a great impact on upper-body strength. But, triathlon swim training gives your all-over fitness an almighty boost. Swimming for triathlon requires even greater upper-body strength than standard swimming, as your objective on race day will be to conserve as much leg strength as possible. Expect to see your triceps, biceps and shoulder muscles emerge as you train.

9 It'll make you better at everything We're not being facetious. Each discipline in triathlon supports the others, so, for example, runners who increase swim training often report improvements in their running, too. This is because swimming is a fantastic way to build core stability, which is crucial for good running form. Likewise, cycling promotes your endurance for swimming and running.

10 It'll boost your bone strength Weight-bearing exercise, such as running, is a great way to boost your bone density, which is particularly important for women. Osteoporosis is increasingly common in young as well as older women owing to the fact that our activity levels in the UK have decreased in recent years, while we're also eating less dairy produce (needed for healthy bone development and maintenance). What's more, if you include the resistance workout we have created specifically to complement your triathlon training (see page 164) you'll be doing your bones even more of a favour, as working out with weights has bone-building benefits.

What's stopping you?

Tempted to start tri training, but put off by some niggling worries? We've got them covered.

The worry: 'Isn't it a bit nerdy?'
Says who? Triathlon is the UK's fastest-growing sport, and one of the fastest-growing sports in the USA, Australia and South Africa. The thousands of people who competed in triathlon races last year can't all be nerds, surely? The kit has improved in leaps and bounds since the sport first took off in the 1980s and 1990s, and there is no shortage of stylish gear out there, if you know where to look. It's sociable, too; there are triathlon training clubs everywhere from Newcastle to Newquay.

The worry: 'I get out of breath after 10 minutes of running – I could never do a triathlon!'
We've done our research, and it's genuinely possible to go from virtual non exerciser to Super-Sprint competitor in 10 weeks. It's basically a question of building up gradually, and balancing your training across the three disciplines. Our Super-Sprint plan (see page 148) is designed with plenty of rest periods, so you'll be able to catch your breath when you need to. You might only be out of breath because you're running too fast. With our training plans, you'll learn to pace yourself.

The worry: 'I don't want to fork out a fortune for something I'm not sure I'll enjoy'
You don't have to spend a fortune, especially not when you start training. In fact, if you already go to the gym now and then, chances are you already have most of what you need. Here's the list: a swimsuit, goggles, shorts and sweat-wicking T-shirt, trainers, for women a sports bra, bike and helmet. There is no need to buy a new bike, wetsuit or other triathlon-specific kit until you are sure you want to carry on. In any case, you can hire a wetsuit for a whole season, or for a weekend.

The worry: 'I'm frightened of open-water swimming'
Don't let this fear put you off. There are plenty of triathlons with pool-based swims to choose from. But if there's a race you want to do with an open-water swim, a few simple tips and training sessions can build your confidence. You won't need to do much open-water training, particularly if you're not aiming for a set race time, and if it's the hordes of other swimmers that worry you, start at the back or side of the pack to avoid knocks.

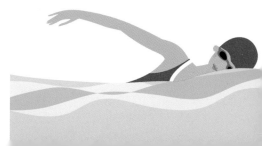

The worry: 'I can't swim front crawl'

You're not alone. In a recent sprint triathlon we entered, a good 30% of competitors were swimming breaststroke. It's perfectly possible to complete your swim in a respectable time without swimming crawl. It's worth being aware though, that swimming breaststroke in a wetsuit is hard work, but the good news is that the added buoyancy that a wetsuit gives you makes swimming crawl a whole lot simpler, and speedier. Bear in mind too, that the swim is the shortest leg of the race, so you can easily make up your time with a stronger cycling and running performance.

The worry: 'I'm not confident on a bike'

Particularly if you live in a city and ride only rarely, starting a cycle-training programme can seem intimidating. But getting over your fears could really change your life. Cycling all, or part of your way to work and back can form the basis of your cycle training, and it saves money, and often time, too. Or find a cycle route near you; these are often on disused railways and are flat and easy to follow. By knowing the rules of the race, and not trying to push ahead, there's no danger of being knocked off by other cyclists. Confidence comes quickly with practice.

The worry: 'Running's hard enough on its own, let alone after a swim and cycle!'

It isn't surprising that this aspect of triathlon puts novices off – it's difficult to adjust to combining the three disciplines. But think of it this way: when you go to the gym, you might spend 10 minutes on the rower, 15 on the running machine, 10 on the cross trainer and another 10 on the bike and think nothing of it. This is the outdoor equivalent, and if you follow our plans, we guarantee you should have plenty of energy to complete the run at the end of the race. There are tactics triathletes employ to make the transitions easier, too (see page 134).

The worry: 'I don't fancy a soggy cycle' In our experience, this is one of the most frequently voiced worries about triathlon. But here's the deal. Firstly, you'll be so focused on the race, you won't even think about the dampness. Secondly, technical kit dries really quickly, particularly as you will be warm. Finally, if you choose to, pulling on a dry pair of shorts over your swimsuit will absorb some of the moisture.

The worry: 'Isn't triathlon training really time consuming?' This is probably the main reason more people don't sign up for a triathlon, but it's a myth that triathlon training has to take over your life. It's perfectly possible to complete a Super-Sprint triathlon training for three hours a week. And there are plenty of ways to reduce the amount this eats into your spare time – you could run or cycle to the pool or to work. Think about swimming or running in your lunch break.

The worry: 'I'll finish the race with wet hair looking dreadful!' This is one of the unspoken worries many women have about the sport. We say there's no shame in a little vanity, particularly when your friends and family will be in the crowd on race day. It is a challenge to look attractive when you emerge from a swim, with goggle marks, zero make-up and straggly hair, but don't let this put you off! *Zest*'s beauty editor, Alexandra Friend suggests waterproof mascara, a slick of Vaseline on your lips, and a hair band to keep your hair off your face (wear it

under your helmet for the cycle, so it's in place for your run). Or take a leaf out of many a female triathlete's book and wear your hair in a French plait. You could also put on a hat and sunglasses for the run, so you finish looking presentable!

The worry: 'I don't want to spend each leg worrying about the next part of the race' If you have done enough training, you won't need to worry. Most triathletes have a stronger, or weaker discipline, so it's natural that one aspect of the race might cause you more worry than others, but the key is to stay calm, and focus on the task in hand. Thinking about the next stage of the race can actually help you to an extent – there are ways you'll need to modify your swimming or cycling technique for example, as you near transition in order to make the changeover easier. For more ideas on this, see page 134.

The worry: 'The thought of doing three different disciplines on an unfamiliar race course terrifies me!'

Although you shouldn't be terrified, it's sensible to find out as much as you can about the course before race day. If it isn't possible for you to go and look at it, don't panic. Most race organisers provide information on the course in advance, so make sure you read it word for word. Building your confidence in every aspect of your training will help too – make sure you've practised open-water swimming before your race if that's what you've signed up for, and if the course is hilly, ensure you've done some hill training. Bear in mind that the course will be clearly marked, there should be marshalls to direct you, and everyone else will be heading the same way.

The worry: 'It's the logistics of switching between sports that puts me off'

To the beginner triathlete, the concept of transition itself is a strange one, and the fact that the clock is ticking can lead to panic. But the secret is planning and practise. Triathlon coaches suggest you think of transition as the 'fourth element' to your race, which sounds scary, but just equates to being well-prepared. The key is to lay out your kit to make sure you can find what you need, and practice the changes at home. See our section on how to do transition.

The worry: 'I'll be the only beginner in a race full of experts'

This is another common worry, but as triathlon is such a growing sport, most races will be packed with other first-timers. To ensure you won't feel out of place, pick a large race or give the organisers a call and ask them if it's beginner-friendly. To give you an indication, the Michelob Ultra London Triathlon (the world's biggest race) had 50% first-timers taking part in 2006! When the day of the race comes, remember to feel proud of yourself just for being there – half of all adults in the UK do no exercise at all, and only one in five do three half-hour sessions a week or more – you're a star!

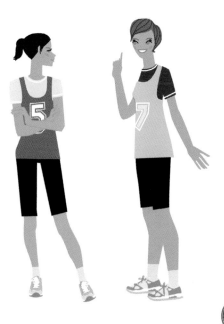

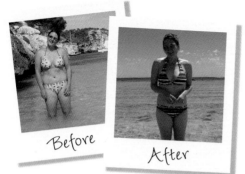

Before

After

Kate Knight, 26,
from Inverness
Height 5ft 3½in

Before
11st 3lb
Dress size 16

After
9st 7lb
Dress size 12

✳ **WEIGHT LOST 1ST 10LB**

'I LOVE BEING FIT AND WOULD NEVER GO BACK'

❝ I had always struggled with my weight and had been on diet after diet since I was 18 – sometimes they worked but I never managed to keep the weight off. In 2005, I eventually decided to try Weight Watchers as it seemed like quite a sensible system of daily points. I had started doing triathlons a year before that, but had been training ineffectively due to my excess weight and eating badly – not bad foods, but just too much of certain groups and very large portions.

Weight Watchers taught me to eat food in a balanced way. I'd have things like toast and banana for breakfast, chicken and salad wraps for lunch and meat and veg for dinner. At the same time, I moved to a new area and joined a triathlon club because I wanted to meet new people and learn how to train properly.

Working out with them totally changed the way I trained by making it much more focused and effective, and the combination of this and my new healthy eating caused the weight I had struggled with for so long to start melting away – the added bonus was that triathlon training meant I could add points to my daily allowance,

which I could use for treats! I was doing one or two swims, one or two runs and one bike ride a week.

I started the diet and training in November 2005 and, by October 2006, I was down from 11st 3lb to my target weight of 9st 7lb. I did a sprint distance race in August 2006, when I was close to my target weight, and knocked 15 minutes off my personal best! For the first time ever, I could see muscle definition on my arms and legs, and my tummy went from wobbly to toned. Tri training with the club also helped me manage the stress of a demanding job – it's a great way to forget all your worries and I made good friends there. I've been this weight for a year now and it's not going back on – I love being fit and would never go back! ❞

Kate's tips
Food: 'Never, ever go hungry. I always carry fruit around with me to satisfy snack cravings.'
Fitness: 'If you have a bad session, don't lose heart and give up. Everybody has off-days!'

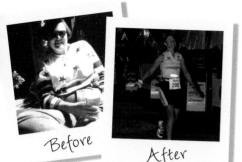

Before

After

**Jenny McGowan, 37,
from Sydney, Australia
Height 5ft 5in**

Before	After
14st 9lb	10st 3lb
Dress size 18	Dress size 10

✳ **WEIGHT LOST 4ST 6LB**

'I WAS A COUCH POTATO – NOW I'M ULTRA-FIT'

❝ Throughout my childhood and teens, I was always quite big, but I didn't yearn to be skinny.

During my 20s, I became a party girl and would be out several nights a week with my husband, drinking creamy cocktails and smoking at least 20 cigarettes a day. I slowly put on more weight until I weighed 14st 9lb.

In 1997, my (now ex-) husband was out of work and we had to have a look at our budget. The cigarettes were first on the list of habits that had to go. I knew that you often put on weight when you quit smoking – so I decided to take up some exercise.

I started off by joining a running group. Years of no exercise made this a tough experience, but I built up from walk/running to running. As I started signing up for races, I became more aware of what I was eating and made changes to my diet. Before, I would cook lots of rich food with cream and wine, but I cut down on that and started eating fresh, unprocessed foods, lean meat and lots of fruit and veg. I also cut right down on alcohol. I lost 1st 8lb in six months.

When I started suffering a foot injury from running, a friend suggested I take up cycling as a way of cross-training. This led to another friend suggesting I try triathlon, so I signed up for a Super-Sprint in 2001. I loved it, so I joined my local triathlon club.

I quickly saw a change from tri training – my body became stronger and more defined, and I lost another 2st 12lb in six months. I became addicted to longer and longer triathlons and, in 2003, I decided to go for an Ironman. I trained for 25 hours a week and did the Sydney Ironman in 2004. It took me 13 hours 38 minutes and I cried with elation when I approached the finishing line and the commentator said, "Jenny McGowan, you are an Ironman!" ❞

Jenny's tips

Food: 'Eat as much fresh food as possible and always eat enough to meet your training needs – I eat plenty of carbs for energy and protein for muscle repair.'

Fitness: 'The morning is a great time to train because it leaves the rest of the day free and you feel energised for the day ahead.'

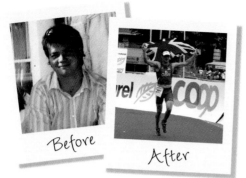

Before

After

**Wil Newbery, 29,
from Hampshire
Height 5ft 9in**

Before	After
13st 7lb	11st 7lb

✳ **WEIGHT LOST 2ST**

'I WENT FROM PARTY ANIMAL TO GREAT BRITAIN TRIATHLETE'

❝ When I left university, I went into marketing and lived a party lifestyle – I ate a lot, drank a lot and was a social smoker. My weight slowly crept to 13st 7lb. Then one day in 2003, my brother-in-law goaded me into doing the London Marathon. Thinking I was sporty because I'd played hockey at school, I agreed and went out for my first run. I almost collapsed after half a mile, had to rest for 10 minutes and came home defeated.

I realised that I would have to make a few radical changes, so gave up smoking, started eating more healthily by cutting out the takeaways and adding in lots of fruit and vegetables, and went teetotal for a few months. I even started to enjoy my training so much that I signed up for a personal-training course!

After four months of training and 7lb lighter, I managed to complete the marathon. I qualified as a personal trainer a week after the race and gave up my job to become a full-time trainer.

After a few months, I wanted a new challenge. My boss suggested doing a triathlon and lent me his bike. I loved the training – I live in the New Forest so went out for long bike rides and runs through the forest. I did my first sprint-distance triathlon in 2003 and loved it so much I decided to take triathlon more seriously.

The triathlon training totally changed my body because I was now using every single part of it. The pounds started dropping off as everything toned up and I started to see real muscle definition.

'Two years and many races later, I'd improved my times so much, I qualified for the ITU Triathlon World Championships in Switzerland! I came 40th overall and am now ranked 8th in the country. Triathlon is a truly great sport – it's exciting and challenging, and the races are really friendly. ❞

Wil's tips
Food: 'Get used to reading the ingredients on food labels. If you can't pronounce them, then put it back on the shelf.'
Fitness: 'Joining a club, whether it's a gym or triathlon club, is a great way to meet new friends with similar hobbies and boost your training.'

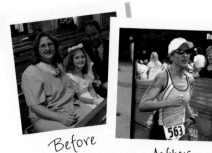

Before

After

Carol Scheible, 44, from North Carolina, US
Height 5ft 6in

Before	After
17st 6lb	9st 9lb
Dress size 24	Dress size 10

✳ WEIGHT LOST 7ST 11LB

'I WAS A FRUMPY HOUSEWIFE, NOW I'M AN ATHLETE'

❝ 'When I was 20, a cousin of mine started doing triathlons. I remember thinking, "that sounds cool, but I could never do that". I was never sporty and considered myself unathletic.

Twenty years later, I was overweight, out of shape and miserable. A combination of having children, no exercise and an addiction to carbs (especially sweets) meant my weight had crept up to 17st 6lb.

One day in 2002, I was at an amusement park with my daughter and we got on a rollercoaster. I couldn't get the strap done up and the attendant came over and used all his might to stretch it around me. I felt so humiliated and resolved to start leading a healthy lifestyle.

I started off by changing what I ate, and got down to just over 13st. Then I hit a plateau. I decided it was time to introduce exercise. I came across a plan online that took you from being a couch potato to running 5K. It was tough because I was overweight and unfit, so I started with walk/running and built up.

All the while, that old thought about triathlon kept resurfacing. This time, instead of thinking "I can't do it"; I thought "I will do it!" so I added biking and swimming to my workouts. The exercise proved to be the key to my final stage of weight loss and I lost another 50lb in a year through training.

In 2005, at 42, I completed my first triathlon. I've done nine more and am fitter than I've ever been in my life! It doesn't take athletic ability, speed or a lean body to be a triathlete. All it takes is setting a goal and persistence in doing whatever it takes to reach that goal.

Triathlon has changed me in many ways. My body shape has changed and I have more energy. I used to be a frumpy housewife, now I'm an athlete. ❞

Carol's tips
Food: 'If I was tempted by unhealthy snacks, I'd have a cup of tea! The milk and small amount of sugar was enough to take the edge off my snack craving and the warm drink was comforting.'
Fitness: 'Setting goals is definitely the key. Sign up to a race to give you a reason to exercise.'

It isn't only your body that'll benefit from triathlon training. It will boost your confidence and ability to focus, and slash your stress levels, too. We explain why.

2
the mood makeover

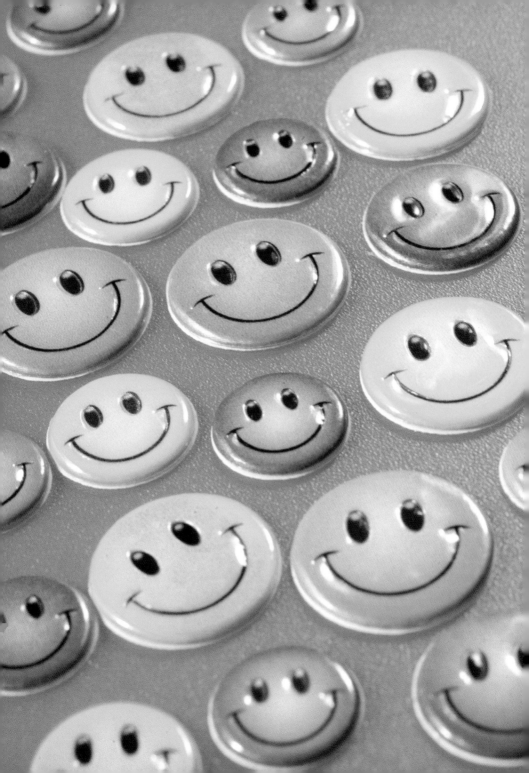

Serenity, success and better sex!

There are so many good reasons to train for a triathlon; a new improved body and an amazing sense of achievement just for starters! Here are some more to help keep you motivated.

You get to feel like a star

If you've ever competed in a running race, you'll know just how fantastic it feels when there are crowds of strangers (and hopefully a few friends or family, too) cheering you on. With all the support, and then the event photographers poised to take your picture at the end, you'll get a real buzz from the attention. 'One of the things I love most about competing in triathlons is how proud of myself it makes me feel,' says 32-year-old Sally Beaumont. 'I'm a mum of two with a sensible job, so it's great to have a bit of glory every now and then!'

You'll be at one with the elements

Even if you've been a confirmed indoor exerciser in the past, you'll fall in love with the great outdoors as a consequence of your triathlon training. Running through the park, along a riverbank, or on the beach beats exercising in the gym every time.

'Once you've felt the wind on your face as you climb to the top of a hill on your bike and take in the view, or got to the halfway point in your first open-water swim, surrounded by fresh water, trees and even the occasional fish, the gym is sure to lose some of its appeal,' says keen triathlete Sam Hayward. Swim coach Helen Gorman maintains that open-water

swimming is exercise 'as it's meant to be – the natural setting makes it so much more pleasurable'.

You'll have more sex

It's official – getting fit will almost certainly have a positive effect on your sex life. Research from the Harvard School of Public Health revealed that men who exercised vigorously for 20–30 minutes a day were half as likely to have erection problems as their sedentary counterparts. Likewise, researchers at the University of Texas measured the sexual responses of 35 women who watched an erotic film with and without a prior session of vigorous cycling. They found that blood flow to the genital tissues had increased while arousal was boosted 169% after exercise.

You'll relax and chill out

If you're the type of person who internalises stress and tends to worry about work, family and relationship pressures more than you should, triathlon training will take you out of a negative-thought cycle.

The physical acts of swimming, running and cycling are some of nature's best mind-clearers. Fran MacDonald, 29, a banker from London, says tri training is her alternative to therapy: 'I love the rhythmic feeling of hitting the pool after a nightmare day at work – it's as if I'm swimming out of all the stress and pressure of the past 24 hours – my brain simply won't let me worry any more.'

The reduction in cortisol and the boost of endorphins (the body's own feel-good hormones) you get during exercise will leave you feeling better able to cope, and with a renewed sense of perspective, too.

It'll encourage you to aim high

Setting yourself a challenge of finishing a triathlon will benefit your approach to life and work. As life coach Pete Cohen says: 'Completing your first triathlon will give you a fresh incentive to set targets in other areas of your life. It's a question of getting into the habit of "daring" yourself to try something outside of your comfort zone. The snowball effect will make you feel more fulfilled and increase your confidence when it comes to going for that promotion at work, or signing up for that class you've been considering.'

You can help to make the world a better place

If you swap some of the journeys you usually make by public transport for commuting by bike or on foot, you'll reduce your environmental footprint, which should give you an altruistic buzz. If you sign up for a race, you can take it one step further and get sponsored for any good cause that's close to your heart. The benefit goes both ways – knowing you're doing a triathlon with a purpose will spur you on when your motivation is waning.

You'll learn to love your body

Very few people are 100% confident with their body. Even the superfit have complaints. But there's nothing quite like knowing your body is strong enough to get you through a race to make you feel positive about the shape you're in.

It's also good to know you could swim, run or cycle your way out of danger if ever you needed to. Triathlon training inspires you to develop the kind of all-round fitness that most people only dream about. As you see your newly defined waist and arm muscles emerging, and feel your bottom getting smaller and tighter, you'll know you've done it the healthiest way possible.

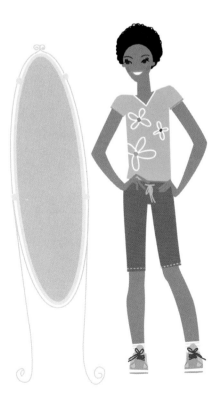

The joy of tri

Triathlon training and competing can have some fantastic side effects. We asked a range of triathletes what they love most about the sport...

'I'm loving the training for my first tri. I've done a few 5K races before, and decided to put myself down for a Super-Sprint when my gym regime got boring. I'm feeling fitter than I have in years, and I'm really enjoying my gorgeous ride to work every morning – it means I arrive at my desk feeling really positive – ready for anything the day might throw at me. I signed up when my super-sporty flatmate said she was planning a tri. I know she'll beat me, but being competitive, she really inspired me to give it a go.'
Rebecca Williams, age 32

'The thing I love most about triathlon is that it's still relatively untouched as a sport, and people have a great deal of respect for triathletes. If you say you're a runner, people think "Great, but who isn't?" But if you say you're a triathlete, there's a whole different level of respect. Training for triathlons gives you a sense of achievement and wellbeing like no other discipline. It also makes you more in tune with your body and mind. I've learnt to listen to the subtle messages my body sends out, and heed them.' **Tim Barber, age 40**

'I'll be forever grateful to triathlon for introducing me to open-water swimming. I loved the training, particularly the long swims – I'd cycle to London's Tooting Lido every Sunday, and swim for 40 minutes. I also signed up to join a running club as part of my training which was hugely motivating. I dropped 10lb and developed lots more muscle definition. Although the swim on race day was a bit of a scrum, it inspired me to set up an outdoor swimming society!'
Kate Rew, age 38

'In my life I have very little opportunity to be alone with my thoughts. Running and swimming are both really meditative, and the only way I can let my mind drift. I had always assumed triathlons were extremely difficult before I tried one, but I found that I enjoyed it, and it was a lot easier than I'd imagined. Training is the perfect excuse to explore beautiful places, whether that's a local park, forest or river.' **Jeremy Beament, age 29**

'I signed up for my first triathlon after completing a number of marathons and feeling I needed a new goal. What surprised me most was how much I enjoyed the swimming. I'd never been able to swim front crawl in the past, but through my triathlon training I surprised myself by enjoying it. Having said that, I did bottle out on race day and swim breaststroke, but that didn't matter – I'd learnt a new skill! Now I've completed a few triathlons, and I love it. What's unique about triathlon is the way it allows people with different strengths all to race together. My friend is a really excellent swimmer and great on a bike, while I'm a good runner. It means I can spend the whole triathlon chasing after her then we can battle it out during the run. The competition brings out the fighting spirit in both of us!' **Susie Whalley, age 34**

'I did my first tri in 2002, having previously competed only in running races. I was amazed at the cross-section of people taking part. Tall, short, large, small, young and old. The array of bikes ranged from carbon-fibre Lance Armstrong-worthy machines to 1980s mountain bikes and shoppers. I thought that was fantastic. The race was tough, particularly the run (my legs didn't feel like they were mine) but as I collapsed into my girlfriend's arms at the finish, a wave of euphoria kicked in. I was hooked!' **Ian Lowe, age 49**

'I've met some great friends through triathlon training, and more than anything else, I really enjoy it. Even if I come last in a race, I figure that I beat everyone who didn't take part. I love the fact that I'm always racing against myself, and really enjoy the beautiful locations I train in, too.' **Linda Connor, age 42**

'I love the variety that triathlon training offers. If it's pouring with rain, a trip to the local pool is on the cards, while a fabulous sunny weekend means a bike ride is great fun. There's never an excuse not to train – even when I'm short of time, a fast run works well. If I have sore legs from running, I'll hit the pool for some arm work. I used to think of it as a sport for the elite, but it's the most inclusive sport imaginable. Everyone has their strengths and works hard to race to them.'
Sara Beazley, age 39

The joy of tri

'When I trained for running alone, it was all about getting the mileage and speed training in every day. With triathlon training I don't get bored and I can swap the sessions around to suit my mood. It's more sociable, as I can train for the different sports with different friends. I love the way it gives you an all-over body workout. There's always something to improve, whether it's one of the three disciplines, your transition time, or your speed.'
Lindsay Cunningham, age 34

'I did my first triathlon ten years ago. The swim was in a pool, I rode a mountain bike and the only thing I can remember about the run is having a terrible stitch, but I kept going and felt a huge sense of achievement as I crossed the finish line. I discovered later that I'd come third in my age group! Since then I've grown to really enjoy the training – I love going for long rides on my super-shiny road bike, and never get bored.' **Alison Hamlett, age 34**

'After finishing my first Ironman, in Florida, I was asked to give a presentation to my son's fourth-grade class about my race. I worked out that the distance I'd travelled in that race (140.6 miles), was further than the distance from Philadelphia to Baltimore – that impressed me. Reflecting on what I'd achieved, I realised I'd fulfilled a dream I'd believed impossible five years ago. No other accomplishment, amount of money or trophy could ever make me feel as proud as I did at that moment! The essence of triathlon is that no matter where you are in the field (front of the pack, middle of the road, or back), there's a personal challenge to overcome. Unlike in any other sport I've tried, all the triathletes I've met really appreciate and respect one another's strengths.' **Andy Rosebrook, age 37**

'I love copying out my tri training programme into my diary and knowing I'm going to be run-, bike- and swim-fit in the space of a few months. I love all the kit, too! Simply looking at my wetsuit and bike inspires me to go out training. Swimming in my local lido in the morning or getting to work having cycled 5K and swum 1K all before 9am makes me proud! My proudest moment was standing around at the start of the Michelob Ultra London Triathlon in my wetsuit with all the competitors. I thought to myself, "You know what? I'm a triathlete now!"' **Jess Spring, age 31**

'I've always considered myself a relatively fit person, but until recently was more of a gymgoer than a competitive type. That all changed in October 2005, when I qualified as a personal trainer and wanted to set myself another goal to achieve in 2006. After reading an article about different ways to fundraise, I thought I'd try a triathlon. I was worried that at 42 I was a bit old. But I fell in love with the sport and now I look forward to setting myself training and race goals for the year to come. I get a real buzz from knowing that at 43, I'm fitter than I've ever been before. Triathlon has taught me that if I set my mind to pretty much anything, I can achieve it! It's made me more positive and fearless in every area of my life.' **Audrey Livingston, age 43**

'The best thing that's come out of my tri training is the friends I've made. I also love the focus that triathlon gives me. The build-up is just as much fun as the race. Planning key training sessions, finding new cycle routes, entering new running races in the build-up to a major triathlon is all part of what makes it so enjoyable. Every season is different, too, as I make sure I'm always trying new races. My most memorable tri moment was finishing my first Ironman in Austria in 2005. It was the culmination of a challenging six months, and I felt very emotional crossing the finish line. Triathlon has made me realise how much my body and mind is capable of!' **Andrea Sullivan, age 31**

'My family joke that when I'm moody, I just need to go out training, and I'll come back 100% better. I love being outdoors, sweating, working hard, and focusing intently on a single goal. I love the challenge of triathlons. There is always a skill to be learnt, an objective to reach, and a discipline to improve. I read an article that summed up why I love to train so much – it talked about the sense of peace that comes in a training session. It's as if the world is on hold, and I can simply focus on myself. Training helps me to understand myself better.' **Kelly Couch, age 29**

'I discovered open-water swimming through training for a triathlon, and realised that as a competitive swimmer spending hours training in the pool, I'd been missing out on a whole other world of swmming. When I'm swimming in a lake, I feel it's how swimming really should be – I love being able to look around at the trees and ducks – it's like the difference between running on a treadmill and running outside.' **Helen Gorman, age 35**

○ ○ ○ On top of the feel-good buzz
that comes from completing
your first triathlon, we're
betting that at least part of
your motivation is physical.
If so, you've picked the right
sport. We believe there's
no better way to transform
your body than through tri
training. Want to know why?

3
the body
benefits

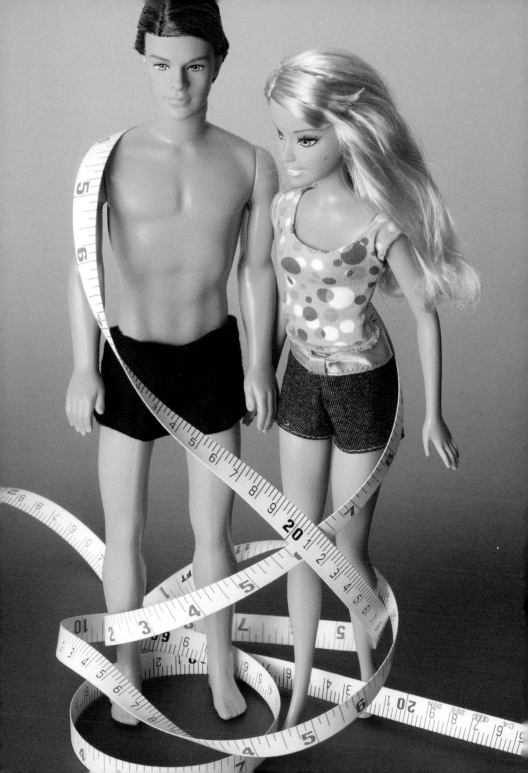

Our promise to you

Before we get started, we want to tell you exactly what to expect from the training plans in this book and the advice we offer. We wrote *Triathlon Made Easy* because we couldn't find a book out there that really took triathlon back to basics; the books we cound find assumed that the reader had a fair degree of fitness or knowledge already.

We promise that our plan makes no such assumption. If you are new to exercise or triathlon, the Super-Sprint plan is designed with you in mind. The stop-start approach featured in the plan enables you to build up gradually.

WE PROMISE to help you overcome your fears

If you're already fairly fit, but nervous about one or more aspects of triathlon training, our skill-specific pointers will offer the advice you need to get you on track. For example, if you've run a few 10K races and feel confident in the swimming pool, but you're terrified of cycling on the road, the cycling chapter will take you right back to basics, advising you on everything from the perfect seat height to how to keep safe on the road when you're training. The same goes for those of you who aren't enthusiastic about getting wet (and yes, that even applies if you currently swim breaststroke with your head above the water!).

WE PROMISE to motivate you along the way

We'll help you to fall in love with every aspect of triathlon, and to look forward to the post-training euphoria – whatever discipline you've been working on that day. Built into the programme are daily, weekly and long-term rewards to keep you motivated, and our journal section (designed for you to fill in) contains inspiring thoughts to help keep you going.

WE PROMISE that this won't take over your life

Unless you want it to, of course! Our sessions have been designed around the fact that every triathlete needs a life outside of training. Each of our 10-week training programmes (see Tri in Ten plans, page 144) is guaranteed to ensure you are well prepared on race day, without demanding too much of your time, or body.

WE PROMISE that you won't ever be bored

The plans are efficient, varied and achievable, which means you won't get bored or frustrated. Ready to dig out those trainers?

Hands up if you'd like...

- A slimmer stomach
- To stop worrying about your weight
- Firm thighs
- Sculpted shoulders
- Greater lung capacity
- To feel confident on the beach
- Cheekbones you can see and no double chin
- A healthier heart
- Glowing skin
- A firm bottom
- Taut, toned arms with no wobble
- Less body fat and better muscle tone
- Honed hips
- To borrow your skinny friend's clothes
- To say goodbye to fat days
- To challenge your child to a race and win!
- A longer life

ADD YOUR OWN:

_____

_____

_____

_____

_____

If you've answered 'yes' to all, or most, of the above, it's time to get excited! Your body is about to undergo the transformation of a lifetime.

Sticking with it: the secrets

What is it that enables some people to follow a training regime to the letter, while others start out keen, then let negativity get the better of them? A few simple changes in your approach and attitude can make all the difference.

Be realistic

If you're the type of person who gets carried away with a new sport, hobby or goal then tires of it equally quickly, watch yourself. Don't pick an advanced training plan for the sake of it, and don't expect to find the training easy at once. The whole point of training for a triathlon is that your fitness, skills and confidence improve over the weeks. Enjoy the journey, and don't get disheartened if you have to stop for a rest now and then, or intersperse your running with walking breaks. Being overly hard on yourself will only backfire when you fail to live up to your own high standards.

Keep it varied

To an extent, we've done the hard work for you with our Tri in Ten plans (see page 144) – all three programmes are very varied – so you won't feel you're always doing the same training session. The skill drills in each of our sections will ensure you have plenty to focus on as you train, too. In addition to this, vary your training locations as much as you can.

If you're going away for a weekend, pack your trainers, or take your bike. Seek out new routes near your home, and visit different pools. If you like, train at different times of the day, too.

Think bite-sized goals

Don't rely on race day as your sole goal. 'The more mini targets you can build into your training, the better,' says Midgie Thompson, a mental performance coach. 'Whether it's beating your time on a set running or cycling route, losing 5lb within a fortnight, or rediscovering your biceps thanks to your swim training, keeping a mental list of achievements ensures there is always something to celebrate.' Log them in your diary at regular intervals so you have plenty to tick off! That way, if one aspect of your training isn't going so well, you won't get disheartened.

Tailor your training

'Don't follow a training plan on auto-pilot,' says Thompson, who is surprised by the number of athletes (both amateur and professional) she sees who don't consider adapting their training to suit their personality. 'If you find running on a treadmill mind-numbingly dull, don't plan a gym-based brick session [going straight from one discipline to the next].' Or if you don't relish the pool, try an outdoor swim. 'It's important to remember that your aim is to enjoy your training – a fact that many novice triathletes forget. Don't be too rigid and beat yourself up just because you didn't do exactly as the training plan indicated.'

Have a contingency plan

If it's pelting down with rain, don't give yourself an excuse to kick back and spend the night in front of the TV. Always have a plan B at the back of your mind. Do a spinning class instead, focus on some core conditioning at home (use the exercises on pages 162–3), or try some body conditioning moves (see pages 164–5). If the bikes and treadmills are all in use in the gym, spend 15 minutes on the cross-trainer or rower. View the problem as an opportunity to try something new; you'll still be training the right muscles, but in a different way.

Dare yourself

If your motivation is flagging, and you find yourself running through a series of excuses as to why you don't need to train, practise the '10-minute rule'. Tell yourself you'll try to swim, run or cycle for just 10 minutes, then if you really want to, you can stop. Once you've begun, you'll probably want to carry on. The toughest part of motivation is getting past the door, but this simple trick can work wonders when you're not in the mood.

Change your focus

'One of the biggest traps novice triathletes fall into is that they get stuck in a negative-thought cycle that becomes a self-fulfilling prophecy,' according to Tom Breeze, a sports psychology consultant who specialises in motivation. 'If you spend a training session thinking "This is hard work, my legs feel heavy, I'm tired", you're making the session even harder for yourself.'

Instead, Breeze suggests making a conscious effort to focus on other sensations, whether that's by listening to the sound of children playing in the park, or running through the words to a favourite song in your head. You could even focus on another part of your body that feels energetic or relaxed. This will help you to 'zone out' of the discomfort and enjoy the session more.

Spread the word

Time and again, people who embark on a healthy eating and exercise regime make the same mistake – keeping quiet about their ambitions. If you tell other people about an event you are training for, you'll be strengthening your own resolve to complete every training session. When you know your colleagues will be asking you how your training is going, it's an incentive to keep on top of it. The more people you can get behind you, the better. Ask your partner, family, friends and work mates for support, and tell them about your training (and weight loss, if that's what you're aiming for).

Go somewhere

If you have a demanding job and home life, triathlon training can feel like added pressure – which is *so* not the point! If you're feeling under pressure, consider adapting your training to fit more snugly within your life. Could you cycle to and from work, then get off your bike when you get home and do a 20-minute run? That's your brick session out of the way! Or perhaps you could recruit a friendly colleague to join you on a lunchtime run – having another person to spur you on (and ignite your competitive instinct) could be just the motivation you need.

Don't obsess about speed

This is a common beginner's mistake, particularly if you're the competitive type. The most important thing is that you enjoy your training, particularly for your first triathlon. 'Many people who are new to triathlon set a time goal for race day, and then feel disappointed if they can't meet it,' says Midgie Thompson. This can be a major motivation drain. Instead, Thompson suggests adjusting your goals as your training progresses, and focusing on the pleasure of the journey, rather than how fast you can get from A to B. You can always speed up halfway through the race, when you realise you've got plenty of energy left. And there's always next time!

Create a mind movie

Visualisation can be a powerful way to boost performance, and build confidence before a race. It's simple to do, and will help you to feel prepared and relaxed rather than apprehensive and tense.

Tom Breeze suggests spending 5 minutes before a tough training session, or 10 minutes before a race, closing your eyes and conjuring a mental picture of yourself at each stage of the race. 'Imagine yourself in the water, feeling full of energy and pacing yourself well, then visualise each phase of your transition going without a hitch. On the bike, see yourself with the wind rushing past you, feeling in control, and overtaking slower cyclists. Then, with the bike-to-run transition, imagine feeling strong, and not being fazed by the heaviness of your legs. Focus on the sounds and sights you'll pass on the run, then, finally, imagine yourself sprint-finishing to the sound of the crowd's cheers!'

Build a performance profile

'Doing a mini audit of every aspect of your triathlon fitness is a great way to boost motivation,' says Breeze, 'as it enables you to set a host of mini targets to set to work on.' He suggests you write a list of every quality, personality trait and fitness aspect you need to become the best you can be at triathlon. Rate the importance of each trait out of 10 (depending on how important it is to you achieving your race-day or fitness goals). Next, honestly mark out of 10 where you are on the scale. Keep a log of these markers, and make it your mission to improve your score on as many of them as possible.

Pick a body idol

Think about someone whose physique or athletic ability you really admire. Whenever you feel yourself flagging, ask yourself what they would do in your situation. You could even keep a picture of your inspirational figure stuck to your fridge, or by your desk at work – anywhere you will see it regularly. This should act as a trigger, inspiring you to strengthen your resolve whenever you feel the sofa or local pub calling (you can always reward yourself with a glass or two later!).

Avoid burn-out

Make sure there is plenty of downtime built into your training schedule. Whether that's a yoga class, family walk or dinner with friends, you should always have time for the people and activities that help you feel balanced, happy and rested. And when your training plan tells you to take a rest day, heed the advice. 'When you train, your muscles develop tiny tears, and you deplete your energy stores. In order to replenish those and give your muscles time to recover, it's important to schedule rest, and not to overdo one aspect of your training,' says Bill Black, an Olympic triathlon coach who created our Tri in Ten plans. Warm-downs and stretching are important for the same reason, so don't skip them.

Do it for you

Ask yourself who you are training for. 'Athletes who are always seeking to impress another person (whether it's their parents, partner or coach) are more likely to feel like a failure than those who are training for their own satisfaction and enjoyment,' says Tom Breeze. Stay focused on what *you* are getting out of the training, whether it's a better body, cardiovascular fitness or a real sense of achievement.

'A certain amount of selfishness is crucial when it comes to successful training and competing.'

Spoil yourself

When you're pushing your body, it's important to ensure your body and mind feel nourished and energised, rather than neglected and drained. Sam Naylor, a keen amateur triathlete, says, 'Whenever I'm in training for a big race, I make a pact with myself that I'll keep my fridge stocked with healthy, delicious food and ensure there are fresh flowers in my bedroom and a bottle of my favourite wine in the fridge.' Think about what works for you and makes you feel well looked after. This could be getting a taxi home after a tough day, or treating yourself to a weekly takeaway and DVD. Your training means you deserve it more than ever. For more ideas on how to spoil yourself, turn over the page!

35

MY MISSION STATEMENT

I _____ **(name)** do hereby declare that I am determined to get fit/fitter (delete as appropriate).

The long-term goal that I am aiming for is _____, which I aim to achieve by _____ **(date)**. I have chosen this goal because it will make me feel _____

_____

and enable me to prove that _____.

In order to achieve the goal I've set, I pledge to complete the Tri in Ten training plan best suited to my fitness level. I promise that I'll be firm with myself when it comes to sticking with the training, but kind to myself when I'm on track. I will do this by celebrating with a daily reward chosen from the Daily Rewards list (see opposite). At the end of every week on the programme, I'll celebrate by treating myself to a weekly reward chosen from the Weekly Rewards list (see opposite).

To keep myself motivated, I will cut out a picture showing the body of an athlete, friend or healthy celebrity whom I admire, and look at it every time I find my motivation waning.

If I fail to complete the Tri in Ten training plan, I promise to choose a penalty from the list opposite.

When I reach my goal, I promise to celebrate by spoiling myself with

_____

chosen from the Ultimate Rewards list (see opposite). I also promise to pin this mission statement somewhere I can see it clearly (the fridge, or on the inside of my wardrobe door), and read it as often as possible.

Today's date is _____, and I pledge to complete my long-term goal by _____.

My rewards

Here is the list of rewards that you can choose from when you complete your training. Choose one for every day that you train, at the end of a successful week, and when you achieve your ultimate goal. There are also some 'penalties' for when you need some extra discipline!

Daily rewards
Allow yourself one of these pleasures after every training session:
- Have a long, candlelit bath
- Eat a healthy pudding (we suggest a baked apple stuffed with sultanas, or tropical fruit salad)
- Rediscover an old CD or album you haven't heard in ages
- Retreat to a comfy chair with a book for half an hour
- Sip a cool glass of crisp, white wine
- Try a DIY health or beauty ritual – maybe an invigorating salt scrub, massage or pedicure
- Relax in a soothing Jacuzzi

Weekly rewards
Choose one of these at the end of the week when you've completed all your training sessions:
- Invest in a flattering new swimsuit or pair of cycling shorts
- Read an inspiring magazine
- Go out for dinner, and order whatever you fancy
- Enjoy a languorous lie-in
- Buy a new plant or flowers for your desk or home
- Have dinner while watching your favourite TV programme
- Buy a new item of clothing or shoes that you've been pining for

Ultimate rewards
This is for when you complete your first triathlon or achieve a new goal, such as a personal best, or a new distance:
- Book yourself a holiday somewhere hot to show off your new body
- Take your partner to dinner at a Michelin-starred restaurant
- Try something you've always dreamed of, such as trapeze, horse-riding or a flying lesson
- Buy the new bike you now know you will use
- Open a bottle of vintage Champagne to toast your success
- Spend the day in a chic hotel spa for some serious pampering
- Book a box at the opera
- Treat yourself to membership of a cool new gym

Potential penalties
If you know you need an extra motivational push, why not keep one of these on stand-by in case you skip a training session:
- No pudding, all week
- Give up wine for a month
- Volunteer to clean up after your partner for a week
- Spend Saturday afternoon sorting out your sock drawer
- Do without your morning cappuccino all month
- Schedule an extra check-up with your dentist

Before you embark on a training plan, it's important to establish your starting point. We've selected a series of key fitness tests that you can use to chart your progress from now, right through our training programmes and beyond as you get fitter and firmer.

4

take the tests

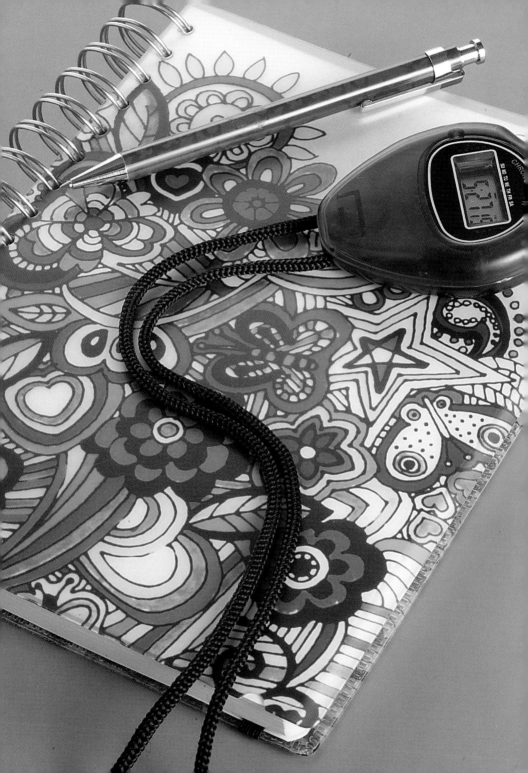

How fit are you?

Here are five key tests to assess your fitness before you get started. Repeat the tests regularly to measure your progress.

Test 1: your heart rate

This is a good test of your cardiovascular fitness. The stronger your heart is, the fewer the number of times it will need to pump per minute to send blood around your body.

Take your pulse first thing in the morning, before you have consumed any stimulants such as caffeine or nicotine and before you have done any kind of physical exercise. Sit down somewhere quiet for a few minutes before you take your pulse.

1. Count the number of beats you can feel at your wrist during a 15-second period.
2. Multiply this number by 4 to get your BPM (beats per minute).

If you want a really accurate figure, take your pulse every day for a week, then work out the average.

Assessing the results

The healthy range for BPM is fairly wide. Anything between 60 and 80 BPM is normal. Athletes and the very fit tend to have a heart rate of between 40 and 60. If your pulse is over 100, you should visit a doctor immediately, as you may be suffering from an abnormally elevated heart rate, which could be dangerous. Likewise, if your rate is under 40, you should also get checked out.

What difference will triathlon training make?

If you are currently unfit, it should make a big difference. Training regularly should lead to a drop in heart rate by one or two beats per minute every fortnight or so. After six months of training, you should expect to see a drop of between 10 and 15 beats per minute. However, no matter how fit you get, your heart rate will never drop more than 20 beats. If you're fit already, expect to see only a minimal decrease, if any.

Test 2: your MHR

If you're serious about training, it's worth measuring your maximum heart rate (MHR). You can work this out with an easy sum:

Men: 220 – your age = your MHR
Women: 226 – your age = your MHR.

So, if you are a 30-year-old woman, your MHR will be 196. Once you have this figure, you can use it as a guide for your training. An easy session should take your heart rate to between 60% and 70% of its maximum (equivalent to effort level 6–7 on a scale of 1–10). An aerobic session should be 70–80% of its maximum,

and if you are really pushing it with short, fast-paced intervals, you should be working at 80–90% of your MHR.

Effort levels

If you don't want to buy an expensive heart monitor, yet don't want to keep stopping to take your pulse rate, the best guide is to think in terms of effort level. If you're taking it easy, aim for an effort level of 5 or 6 on a scale of 1–10, or if you're pushing it to the max, aim for level 9 (you shouldn't be able to sustain a level 9 for more than a few minutes). We have used effort levels alongside MHR in all our training sessions and plans, so you'll know how hard you should be working.

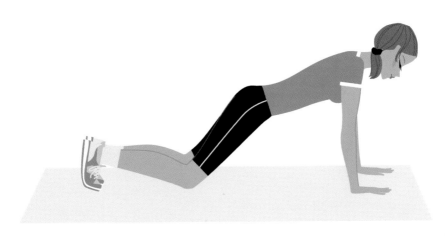

Test 3: your body fat

Your Body Mass Index (BMI) is calculated by dividing your weight (in kilograms) by your height (in metres) squared (see the charts on pages 46–7). But even if you have a healthy BMI, it's always worth checking your body fat percentage.

To get an accurate measurement of your body fat, you will need scales with a body-fat function, found in most gyms. Make sure that each time you measure your body fat, you use the same scales at the same time of day. You need to be naked or in your underwear to get an accurate result.

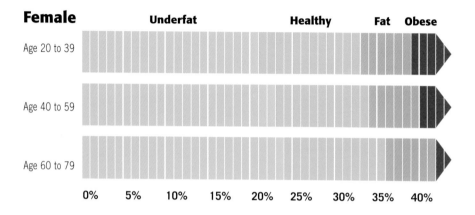

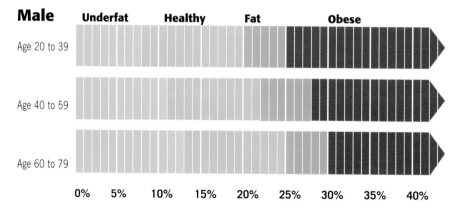

National Institutes of Health/World Health Organisation BMI guidelines, as reported by Gallagher at the New York Obesity Research Center, based on data from the *American Journal of Clinical Nutrition* 2000; 72: 694–701. Data used with permission of the *American Journal of Clinical Nutrition* © Am J Clin Nutr American Society For Clinical Nutrition

Test 4: your flexibility

To measure the flexibility of your back and hamstrings, sit with your legs out straight with your feet resting against a box. Lean forward, measuring how far beyond your toes your fingertips can reach. Hold the reach for two seconds.

20–30cm (8–12in) beyond: very flexible
1–19cm (½–7½in) beyond: average
Not reaching your toes: below average

Tri training can decrease, rather than boost your flexibility, so be sure to do the stretches recommended on pages 60–7 to help maintain flexibility.

Test 5: your leg strength

Your leg strength should improve considerably with triathlon training, so it can be very satisfying to take this test (and note the results) regularly.

Stand with your back against a wall, then lower yourself into a squat position with your thighs parallel to the floor and feet hip-width apart. Hold the position for as long as you can.

Women

46 seconds or longer: very good leg strength
36–45: average leg strength
0–20: poor leg strength

Men

76 seconds or longer: very good leg strength
58–75 seconds: average leg strength
0–30 seconds: poor leg strength

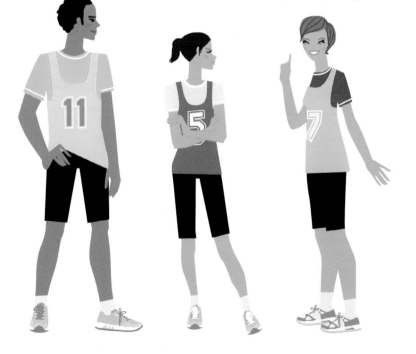

Are you an apple or a pear?

In recent years, a wealth of scientific research has drawn attention to a previously unknown indicator of heart disease, diabetes and cancer risk – the distribution of fat in particular places on the body.

We now know that those who carry a higher proportion of their body fat around their middle ('apple' shape) face more of a health risk than those who carry their fat on the lower half of their body ('pear' shape). So, although your Body Mass Index (BMI) is still an important indicator of your health, your shape is also crucial.

It's helpful to know which camp you fall into. Even if you're not overweight, if you're an apple, it's well worth monitoring your waist measurement and trying to reduce it.

Take the following test:

1. Measure your waist at its narrowest point in centimetres or inches (no breathing in!).
2. Measure your hips at their widest point in centimetres or inches (usually above the pubic line).
3. Divide your waist circumference by your hip circumference.
4. For women, if your score is over 0.8, you're an apple. For men, if your score is over 1, you're an apple. Anything under this is a pear.

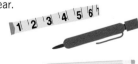

Are you at risk?

A waist measurement greater than 80cm (32in) for women and 94cm (37in) for men is the threshold for increased disease risk.

The greatest risk is for women with a waist measurement of more than 88cm (35in) and men with a waist measurement of more than 102cm (40in).

You're an apple – what now?

The good news is that training for a triathlon is one of the best ways to bring your waist-hip ratio (WHR) down. The exercise will strip excess fat everywhere on your body; and swimming and running are great for blitzing abdominal fat, in particular.

Added to this, the interval training included in our programmes, where you alternate fast bursts of activity with slower-paced recovery intervals, is associated with a significant decrease in abdominal fat.

Doing the core-strengthening exercises (see pages 162–3) will also help to tone the band of muscle that runs around your torso, which supports your spine, pelvis and stomach.

And if you're a pear?

You've struck it lucky in the health stakes, but if you're an overweight pear, you're still at an increased risk of disease, just not such a pronounced one. We're betting that you'd like to rebalance your body shape by slimming down your hips, buttocks and thighs. The Tri in Ten plans will help you to achieve this, with all three disciplines guaranteed to sculpt more shapely thighs, and a firmer bottom. Swimming front crawl in particular (a key part of your training regime) is a great way to slim down hips and thighs.

THE HEALTH BENEFITS OF REDUCING YOUR WAIST

Reducing your waist-hip ratio (WHR) has many benefits; here are just a few highlights:

1. **You'll cut your risk of breast cancer** Women with a WHR over 0.8 are 52% less likely to survive breast cancer than those with a WHR of less than 0.8. Women with high levels of abdominal fat are 45% more likely to develop breast cancer in the first place.

2. **You'll be much less likely to develop diabetes** Women with a waist measurement of 90cm (36in) or more are five times more likely to develop diabetes than their smaller-waisted counterparts. Men with a waist measurement of 102cm (40in) or more are 12 times more likely to develop diabetes.

3. **You'll help your heart** Women with a waist measurement of more than 80cm (32in) were more than twice as likely to suffer a heart attack as those with a smaller measurement.

4. **You'll reduce your blood pressure** Abdominal fat raises your risk of high blood pressure by 60%.

5. **You'll safeguard your brain** One study found that people with high levels of abdominal fat were at a 145% increased risk of developing dementia later in life.

6. **You'll live longer** A man with 1kg (2.2lb) of abdominal fat has double the risk of death compared with a man with half the amount of abdominal fat (½ kg (1.1lb)).

HEALTHY WEIGHT RANGE & BMI TABLE

BMI \ Height	15	16	17	18	19	20	21	22	23	24	25	26	27	28	29	30	31	32	33	34	35
1.47m 4ft 10in	32kg 5st	35kg 5st 7lb	37kg 5st 12lb	39kg 6st 2lb	41kg 6st 6lb	43kg 6st 11lb	45kg 7st 1lb	48kg 7st 8lb	50kg 7st 12lb	52kg 8st 3lb	54kg 8st 7lb	56kg 8st 12lb	58kg 9st 2lb	61kg 9st 9lb	63kg 9st 13lb	65kg 10st 3lb	67kg 10st 8lb	69kg 10st 12lb	71kg 11st 3lb	74kg 11st 9lb	76kg 12st
1.5m 4ft 11in	34kg 5st 5lb	36kg 5st 9lb	38kg 6st	40kg 6st 4lb	43kg 6st 11lb	45kg 7st 1lb	47kg 7st 6lb	49kg 7st 10lb	52kg 8st 3lb	54kg 8st 7lb	56kg 8st 12lb	59kg 9st 4lb	61kg 9st 9lb	63kg 9st 13lb	65kg 10st 3lb	68kg 10st 10lb	70kg 11st	72kg 11st 5lb	74kg 11st 9lb	76kg 12st	78kg 12st 4lb
1.52m 5ft	35kg 5st 7lb	37kg 5st 12lb	39kg 6st 2lb	42kg 6st 9lb	44kg 6st 13lb	46kg 7st 3lb	49kg 7st 10lb	51kg 8st	53kg 8st 5lb	55kg 8st 9lb	58kg 9st 2lb	60kg 9st 6lb	62kg 9st 11lb	65kg 10st 3lb	67kg 10st 8lb	69kg 10st 12lb	72kg 11st 5lb	74kg 11st 9lb	76kg 12st	79kg 12st 6lb	81kg 12st 11lb
1.55m 5ft 1in	36kg 5st 10lb	39kg 6st 2lb	41kg 6st 6lb	43kg 6st 11lb	46kg 7st 3lb	48kg 7st 8lb	50kg 7st 12lb	53kg 8st 5lb	55kg 8st 9lb	58kg 9st 2lb	60kg 9st 6lb	63kg 9st 13lb	65kg 10st 3lb	67kg 10st 8lb	69kg 10st 12lb	72kg 11st 5lb	74kg 11st 9lb	77kg 12st 2lb	79kg 12st 6lb	82kg 12st 13lb	84kg 13st 3lb
1.57m 5ft 2in	37kg 5st 12lb	39kg 6st 2lb	42kg 6st 9lb	44kg 6st 13lb	47kg 7st 6lb	49kg 7st 10lb	52kg 8st 3lb	54kg 8st 7lb	57kg 9st	59kg 9st 4lb	62kg 9st 11lb	64kg 10st 1lb	67kg 10st 8lb	69kg 10st 12lb	71kg 11st 3lb	74kg 11st 9lb	76kg 12st	79kg 12st 6lb	81kg 12st 11lb	84kg 13st 3lb	86kg 13st 8lb
1.6m 5ft 3in	39kg 6st 2lb	41kg 6st 6lb	44kg 6st 13lb	46kg 7st 3lb	49kg 7st 10lb	51kg 8st	54kg 8st 7lb	56kg 8st 12lb	59kg 9st 4lb	61kg 9st 9lb	64kg 10st 1lb	67kg 10st 8lb	69kg 10st 12lb	72kg 11st 5lb	74kg 11st 9lb	76kg 12st	79kg 12st 6lb	82kg 12st 13lb	84kg 13st 3lb	87kg 13st 10lb	90kg 14st 2lb
1.63m 5ft 4in	40kg 6st 4lb	42kg 6st	45kg 7st 1lb	48kg 7st 8lb	50kg 7st 12lb	53kg 8st 5lb	56kg 8st 12lb	58kg 9st 2lb	61kg 9st 9lb	64kg 10st 1lb	66kg 10st 6lb	69kg 10st 12lb	72kg 11st 5lb	74kg 11st 9lb	77kg 12st 2lb	80kg 12st 8lb	82kg 12st 13lb	85kg 13st 5lb	88kg 13st 12lb	90kg 14st 2lb	93kg 14st 9lb
1.65m 5ft 5in	41kg 6st 6lb	44kg 6st 13lb	46kg 7st 3lb	49kg 7st 10lb	52kg 8st 3lb	54kg 8st 7lb	57kg 9st	60kg 9st 6lb	63kg 9st 13lb	65kg 10st 3lb	68kg 10st 10lb	71kg 11st 3lb	73kg 11st 7lb	76kg 12st	79kg 12st 6lb	81kg 12st 11lb	84kg 13st 3lb	87kg 13st 10lb	90kg 14st 2lb	93kg 14st 9lb	95kg 14st 13lb
1.68m 5ft 6in	42kg 6st 9lb	45kg 7st 1lb	48kg 7st 8lb	51kg 8st	54kg 8st 7lb	56kg 8st 12lb	59kg 9st 4lb	62kg 9st 11lb	65kg 10st 3lb	68kg 10st 10lb	70kg 11st	73kg 11st 7lb	76kg 12st	79kg 12st 6lb	82kg 12st 13lb	84kg 13st 3lb	87kg 13st 10lb	90kg 14st 2lb	93kg 14st 9lb	96kg 15st 2lb	99kg 15st 8lb

Healthy weight range (BMI 19–25)

Height

BMI	15	16	17	18	19	20	21	22	23	24	25	26	27	28	29	30	31	32	33	34	35
1.7m 5ft 7in	44kg 6st 13lb	46kg 7st 3lb	49kg 7st 10lb	52kg 8st 3lb	55kg 8st 9lb	58kg 9st 2lb	61kg 9st 9lb	63kg 9st 13lb	67kg 10st 8lb	69kg 10st 12lb	72kg 11st 5lb	75kg 11st 11lb	78kg 12st 4lb	81kg 12st 11lb	84kg 13st 3lb	87kg 13st 10lb	90kg 14st 2lb	93kg 14st 9lb	96kg 15st 2lb	98kg 15st 6lb	101kg 15st 13lb
1.73m 5ft 8in	45kg 7st 1lb	48kg 7st 8lb	51kg 8st	54kg 8st 7lb	57kg 9st	60kg 9st 6lb	63kg 9st 13lb	66kg 10st 6lb	69kg 10st 12lb	72kg 11st 5lb	75kg 11st 11lb	78kg 12st 4lb	81kg 12st 11lb	84kg 13st 3lb	87kg 13st 10lb	90kg 14st 2lb	93kg 14st 9lb	96kg 15st 2lb	99kg 15st 8lb	102kg 16st 1lb	105kg 16st 8lb
1.75m 5ft 9in	46kg 7st 3lb	49kg 7st 10lb	52kg 8st 3lb	55kg 8st 9lb	58kg 9st 2lb	61kg 9st 9lb	64kg 10st 1lb	68kg 10st 10lb	71kg 11st 3lb	74kg 11st 9lb	76kg 12st	80kg 12st 8lb	83kg 13st 1lb	86kg 13st 8lb	89kg 14st	92kg 14st 7lb	95kg 14st 13lb	98kg 15st 6lb	101kg 15st 13lb	104kg 16st 5lb	107kg 16st 12lb
1.78m 5ft 10in	48kg 7st 8lb	51kg 8st	54kg 8st 7lb	57kg 9st	60kg 9st 6lb	63kg 9st 13lb	67kg 10st 8lb	70kg 11st	73kg 11st 7lb	76kg 12st	79kg 12st 6lb	82kg 12st 13lb	86kg 13st 8lb	89kg 14st	92kg 14st 7lb	95kg 14st 13lb	98kg 15st 6lb	101kg 15st 13lb	105kg 16st 8lb	108kg 17st	111kg 17st 7lb
1.8m 5ft 11in	49kg 7st 10lb	52kg 8st 3lb	55kg 8st 9lb	58kg 9st 2lb	62kg 9st 11lb	65kg 10st 3lb	68kg 10st 10lb	72kg 11st 5lb	75kg 11st 11lb	78kg 12st 4lb	81kg 12st 11lb	84kg 13st 3lb	87kg 13st 10lb	91kg 14st 5lb	94kg 14st 11lb	98kg 15st 6lb	101kg 15st 13lb	104kg 16st 5lb	107kg 16st 12lb	110kg 17st 5lb	113kg 17st 11lb
1.83m 6ft	50kg 7st 12lb	54kg 8st 7lb	57kg 9st 4lb	60kg 9st 6lb	63kg 9st 13lb	67kg 10st 8lb	70kg 11st	73kg 11st 7lb	77kg 12st 2lb	80kg 12st 8lb	83kg 13st 1lb	87kg 13st 10lb	90kg 14st 2lb	94kg 14st 11lb	97kg 15st 4lb	100kg 15st 10lb	104kg 16st 5lb	107kg 16st 12lb	110kg 17st 5lb	114kg 17st 13lb	117kg 18st 6lb
1.85m 6ft 1in	51kg 8st	55kg 8st 9lb	59kg 9st 4lb	62kg 9st 11lb	65kg 10st 3lb	69kg 10st 12lb	72kg 11st 5lb	76kg 12st	79kg 12st 6lb	82kg 12st 13lb	86kg 13st 8lb	89kg 14st	93kg 14st 9lb	96kg 15st 2lb	100kg 15st 10lb	103kg 16st 3lb	106kg 16st 10lb	110kg 17st 5lb	113kg 17st 11lb	117kg 18st 6lb	120kg 18st 13lb
1.88m 6ft 2in	53kg 8st 5lb	57kg 9st	60kg 9st 6lb	64kg 10st 1lb	67kg 10st 8lb	71kg 11st 3lb	74kg 11st 9lb	78kg 12st 4lb	81kg 12st 11lb	84kg 13st 3lb	88kg 13st 12lb	92kg 14st 7lb	95kg 14st 13lb	99kg 15st 8lb	103kg 16st 3lb	106kg 16st 10lb	110kg 17st 5lb	113kg 17st 11lb	117kg 18st 6lb	120kg 18st 13lb	124kg 19st 7lb
1.9m 6ft 3in	54kg 8st 7lb	58kg 9st 2lb	62kg 9st 11lb	65kg 10st 3lb	69kg 10st 12lb	73kg 11st 7lb	76kg 12st	80kg 12st 8lb	83kg 13st 1lb	87kg 13st 10lb	91kg 14st 5lb	94kg 14st 11lb	98kg 15st 6lb	101kg 15st 13lb	105kg 16st 8lb	109kg 17st 2lb	112kg 17st 9lb	116kg 18st 4lb	120kg 18st 13lb	123kg 19st 6lb	126kg 19st 12lb
1.93m 6ft 4in	56kg 8st 12lb	60kg 9st 6lb	63kg 9st 13lb	67kg 10st 8lb	71kg 11st 3lb	74kg 11st 9lb	78kg 12st 4lb	82kg 12st 13lb	86kg 13st 8lb	89kg 14st	93kg 14st 9lb	97kg 15st 4lb	101kg 15st 13lb	104kg 16st 5lb	107kg 16st 12lb	112kg 17st 9lb	116kg 18st 4lb	119kg 18st 10lb	123kg 19st 6lb	127kg 20st	130kg 20st 6lb

Healthy weight range (BMI 19–24)

Height

Adapted from a BMI chart supplied courtesy of Weight Watchers (www.weightwatchers.co.uk)

Chart your progress

Whether your goal is weight loss, cardiovascular fitness or more defined muscles, it's important to chart every improvement.

You might find that one week your weight has not changed, but another aspect of your fitness has improved, proving that you're on the way to creating a fitter, stronger body. The chart below should act as inspiration to keep you on target. We recommend that you don't stop training and recording your progress on the last day of the plans in this book. By this point you have shown that you can lead a fit, healthy life. We hope that the three-month and six-month columns inspire you to keep up the good work!

The test	Now	After 2 weeks	After 4 weeks	After 7 weeks	After 10 weeks	After 3 months	After 6 months
Weight							
BMI							
Body fat							
Resting heart rate							
Flexibility							
Leg strength							

Vital statistics

If one of your aims is to lose weight, we recommend that you keep track of your changing body and vital statistics by using a tape measure. Over time you'll have a record of how your body is toning up and improving. Use this page to record your progress.

Top tip

Ensure you take your measurements at the same time of day to achieve consistency; first thing before breakfast is best.

The test	Now	After 2 weeks	After 4 weeks	After 7 weeks	After 10 weeks	After 3 months	After 6 months
Thigh circumference (fullest point)							
Hips at widest point							
Waist at narrowest point							
Upper-arm circumference							

○ ○ ○ Itching to get to the pool, or lace up your trainers? Great. Before you get started, get the lowdown on exactly what kit you'll need, and how to warm up properly and avoid injury. We also reveal our exclusive yoga-based stretch programme designed specifically for triathletes.

5
ready, get set

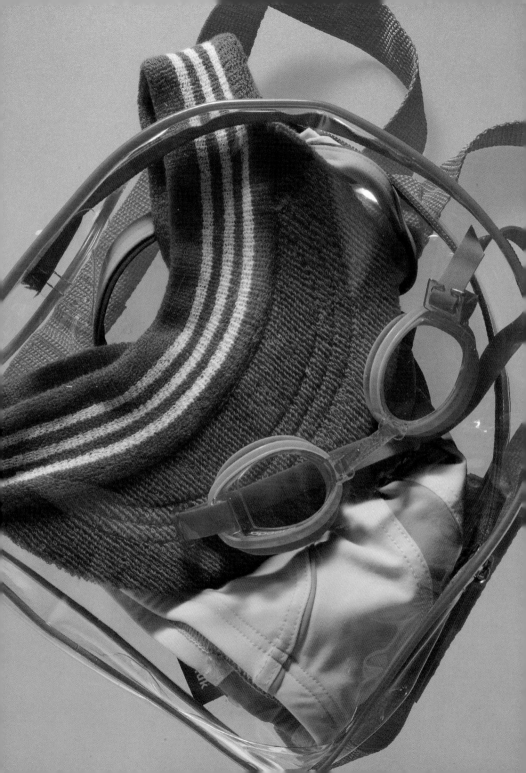

Essential kit to get started

One of the most common assumptions about triathlon is that the kit costs a fortune. This is a myth, particularly when you're starting out.

First things first

There are actually very few items of kit you need to get started, and it's likely that you have all, or most, of them already. Don't worry that you'll look like an amateur in a sea of ultra-professional triathletes with state-of-the-art equipment – any triathlon event that welcomes beginners will be mixed – you won't be the only competitor who is improvising on the kit front.

The biggest potential expense is a bike, but if you have one that's in working order, it doesn't matter if it's a mountain bike or a road bike, as long as you're comfortable riding it. You don't need to buy a new bike, or a bike that is specifically designed for triathlon.

What to wear

Specialist shops sell triathlon suits, which come either as an all-in-one, or as a more flattering vest and shorts set. These are designed to be worn for every phase of the race, including under a wetsuit if you're doing an open-water swim.

If you are entering your first triathlon, you may not want to incur the expense of a triathlon suit, but it saves a lot of hassle on the day, and you won't regret the investment.

Alternatively, you need to wear something that you can run and cycle in, and that you can put on over your

Basic checklist

✓ Bike
✓ Helmet
✓ Trainers
✓ Swimsuit
✓ Goggles
✓ Swimming cap
✓ T-shirt and shorts or a triathlon suit
✓ Cold-weather kit
✓ Socks
✓ Hat
✓ Supportive underwear
✓ Water bottle

swimsuit. If you plan to put on dry clothes after the swim, do bear in mind that any nudity will result in disqualification! Make sure your swimsuit is comfortable enough to cycle and run in.

Wear a sports bra underneath your swimsuit, or select a triathlon suit or tankini with hidden support that's firm enough to keep you secure during the cycle and run.

Swimming kit

Investing in good swim kit will make your training more comfortable and enjoyable. You can wear the same swimsuit and goggles for training as in a race, giving you time to make sure they fit well.

A good pair of goggles

Choose googles that fit properly and won't leak during the swim. A good pair of goggles won't fog, and will improve your vision and comfort as you swim. Reputable sports shops should be happy for you to try on goggles before you buy.

Check that the seal fits comfortably around your eye socket by holding the goggles up to your face, without putting the strap on, and pushing them around your eye sockets. If they stay put, they'll be a good fit; if they fall off, try another pair. Many triathletes favour a mask instead (see page 93).

A comfortable swimsuit

Your swimsuit should fit well and be easy to move in and supportive. It should not rub or dig anywhere. Choose a swimsuit containing Lycra, which helps to support your body and ensures the suit keeps its shape time after time. Some brands come with a chlorine-resistant, or chlorine-proof, promise. Opt for a sport-specific brand rather than a fashion brand, as it will be more likely to last and perform well.

Check the fit by stretching the straps up towards your ears; you should be able to stretch about 5cm (2in) comfortably. Check that you can move your arms and shoulders easily.

A swimming cap

It is compulsory to wear a swimming cap in most triathlons, and many will provide them to indicate which race you are in. It is therefore a good idea to get used to wearing a cap when you're training.

A swimming cap helps to protect your hair from chlorine and stop goggle straps from snagging in your hair. It also makes you more aerodynamic in the water, and has hygiene benefits, too. Caps keep you warm (you lose most of your body heat through your head) – this is a real bonus when you're swimming in open water.

To ensure your hat fits well and doesn't puff up or leak as soon as you get into the water, check that it fits snugly when pulled down fully. You should feel that your head is firmly gripped by the cap.

To help protect your hair when you're swimming, comb conditioner through the hair before you put your swimming cap on; it will save time in the shower later.

Cycling kit

If you become a keen triathlete, there is a wealth of information about bikes, wheels and other kit, all designed to help enhance your performance. When you're starting out, though, none of this is essential.

A roadworthy bike

There is no need to buy a new bike when you take up triathlon; any functioning bike will do. First, check that it's in good working order; take it to your local bike shop for a service.

To check that the bike is a good fit, sit on it and check that the seat is

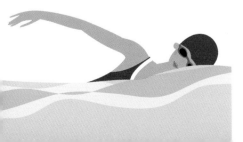

comfortable, and that the frame suits your height and weight. With your feet off the pedals, you should be able to balance on your toes. Place one pedal down at the 6 o'clock position; you should be able to put your heel on the pedal with a straight leg. When the ball of your foot is on the pedal, your knee should have a slight bend in it.

A well-fitting helmet

This a crucial piece of equipment; essential for your safety when training, and vital if you enter a race. You won't be allowed to enter if you don't wear a helmet. To ensure your helmet fits properly:

1. Put it on and do it up under your chin. Adjust the back straps of the helmet so the chin and back strap meets just below your ear lobe. Make sure your chin strap stays in a straight line.

2. Check that you cannot move the helmet so far backwards that your forehead is exposed.

3. Check that you cannot tilt it forward so your eyes are covered.

4. Check that you cannot slide it sideways so one side of your head is uncovered.

When buying a new helmet, make sure it carries a British Standards Kitemark. If yours is old, and you're concerned

about it, take it to your local bike shop for a check. You should replace your helmet if it has a crack in it, or if it has taken a hard knock, even if there are no visible signs of damage.

Shorts and top

If you don't plan to buy a triathlon suit, you'll need a comfortable pair of shorts that you can slip on over your swimsuit, and a cool and comfortable top. Check that the shorts don't have any uncomfortable seams, and ensure they're easy to move in when cycling.

When choosing a top, opt for sweat-wicking fabric. The last thing you want to put on over a swimsuit is cotton.

Women: Make sure you're wearing a supportive tri-suit top or a sports bra underneath your other layers. Running without a supportive sports bra will damage the ligaments that support your breasts. Some brands, such as Shock Absorber, now make a sweat-wicking vest top with inbuilt support.

A water bottle

Staying hydrated is crucial during training, and when you are racing. Invest in a water bottle that can fit inside a bottle cage on your bike and you can use for swimming and running training, too. Ensure it contains enough water (for advice on how much you should be drinking to stay hydrated, see page 71), and that you keep it scrupulously clean.

Wash it with hot water and washing-up liquid after every training session.

Running

The chances are, if you're thinking about training for a triathlon, you already own a pair of running trainers. However, if you plan to increase your training, you may need to check that they're supportive and fit perfectly.

A good-quality pair of trainers

There is no point scrimping when it comes to the shoes you'll be running (and probably cycling) in. Wearing ill-fitting shoes can make you more likely to get injured. It's worth going to a specialist triathlon or running shop, where they can watch you run and help you to select a shoe that's suited to your gait and level of training. Most people overpronate as they run (meaning their feet roll inwards), which can lead to knee and hip problems, but corrective trainers have a dramatic impact. For more information on finding your perfect footwear, see page 131.

A sports bra

You will need a well-fitting supportive sports bra for training, and possibly for race day unless you plan to wear a triathlon suit with inbuilt support. If you do a lot of sport, ensure you change your sports bra regularly (every six months at least) as they lose their elasticity after a while. Ensure your bra is not too restrictive, but makes your chest feel secure and comfortable when you jump up and down.

Shorts and top

If you are not racing in a triathlon suit, you can use the same shorts and T-shirt for cycling and running (and for your training). Opt for synthetic technical fabrics rather than cotton, which can chafe and won't wick away moisture effectively.

Socks

Wearing the wrong socks to train in can cause blisters, and sore, overheated feet. Invest in some properly designed sports socks that have a double layer (the inner encases your foot while the upper layer moves with your trainer) to prevent rubbing. Some triathletes go without socks on race day, but don't do this unless you have tried it before in training!

Cold-weather kit

If you're training in the winter, it's important to keep warm. Most sports brands make full-length tights that are suitable for cycling and running, and will keep your legs insulated. Likewise, investing in a long-sleeved 'base layer' top will keep warmth in, and wick away sweat from your body, while a breathable lightweight jacket (waterproof if you're likely to be training when it's raining) will also be a good investment.

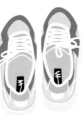

Warming up

When you're pressed for time, warming up can seem unnecessary – why not get straight into the training session? The answer, agree the coaches we spoke to, is that the right sort of warm-up really can reduce your risk of injury and boost your performance during training or a race.

On the flipside, the wrong sort of warm-up can do more harm than good. For example, static stretches, where you stand still and stretch your muscles, which many people still use, have in fact been found to increase risk of injury and decrease muscle strength by up to 20% when performed with cold muscles before a race. They are much better done after training. Instead, warm up by doing 5–10 minutes of the activity you are about to do at a slow pace, then do the dynamic stretches explained here.

The importance of warming up

Whatever you do, resist the temptation to skip a warm-up altogether. 'Going from zero to flat-out is a sure-fire way to increase your chance of getting injured,' says triathlon coach and GB competitor Ralph Hydes. 'For the few minutes you save by not warming up, it really isn't worth the risk.' Pushing 'cold' muscles too hard means they are more likely to get torn, and it increases your chances of suffering from cramp, too.

If you truly don't have time for these stretches every time you train, do at least 5 minutes of the activity you are about to focus on at a gentle pace instead.

For the occasions when you have time for more than a 5-minute warm-up, use the three sequences recommended below (designed by Hydes). 'The dynamic stretches I've recommended should increase joint mobility, and reduce your risk of overstraining,' he says.

How to use the warm-ups

If you are doing just one type of exercise, choose the warm-up for that discipline. If you plan a brick session with cycling and running, use the cycling warm-up before you get started, but go straight from the bike to the run. If you are practising all three disciplines in order (or on race day), many triathlon coaches recommend doing a mini warm-up for all three disciplines in reverse (running, cycling, then swimming), but this isn't always practical. Instead, try a gentle jog, followed by the cycling or running stretches, then some arm rotations to simulate the swimming movement. Keep legs moving as you warm up your upper body.

Swimming

Walk around the poolside or event site for a few minutes to warm your muscles, especially if you have come in from the cold. Before you get into the water, do arm rotations to get the blood flowing to your upper body, and to relax your joints and muscles. If you are doing an open-water swim, the exertion of putting on your wetsuit before you start can act as a mini warm-up in itself before you do the dynamic stretches!

Clockwise arm swings
Stand with your feet hip-width apart, knees relaxed and shoulders down. Swing your arms in wide clockwise arcs for 1 minute.

Anti-clockwise arm swings
Keeping your feet where they are, swing your arms in wide anti-clockwise arcs for 1 minute.

Shoulder rotations
Place both hands on the top of your shoulders. Rotate your upper arms forward, starting with small rotations and getting wider. After 1 minute, rotate your arms backward.

Cycling
Start with 5–10 minutes' easy cycling, in a low gear to allow your muscles to warm up, and to get your legs used to spinning. Then get off your bike and do this stretch routine:

Walking lunges
Lunge on alternate legs as you walk forward. Take care to ensure your knee never bends over your toes, and use the strength from your glutes (buttock muscles) and hamstrings to push you up to a standing position as you complete each lunge. Do five lunges on each side, then switch. Continue for at least 1 minute.

High leg swings
Hold on to a fence or bench with your left hand, and stand side-on to it. Swing your right leg forwards and backwards, getting higher with each swing. Swing slowly, with control, for 1 minute. Repeat on the other side.

Pendulum swings
Stand facing a wall with your arms extended, hands resting on the wall. Swing your right leg in front of your body in a pendulum movement, side to side, 10 times. Again, swing slowly, with control. Return to standing, and then repeat on the other side.

Running
Jog slowly for 5–10 minutes, then try the following dynamic stretches:

Kickbacks
Jog on the spot, attempting to touch your buttocks with your heels. Keep your abs engaged and your pelvis tucked in. Continue for 1 minute.

High knees
Jog on the spot, lifting your knees to waist height as you alternate from foot to foot. Aim to land on your forefoot each time. Keep your arms bent, and pump them as you move. Continue for 1 minute.

Sidesteps
Sidestep for 10 steps at a jogging pace, keeping your weight on the balls of your feet as you move. Allow your arms to swing back and forth as you sidestep and make sure your legs don't cross over. Then sidestep back the other way for 10 steps. Continue for 1 minute.

Avoiding injury

If you are increasing the amount of exercise you do, it's important to protect yourself against injury. Here are a few key pointers to help you avoid getting hurt.

Stay on form

Even if your ambition is simply to complete the course, good form is important to ensure you don't get injured. Your body is designed to work in a certain way, so think about your body position and form as you exercise. Aim to keep a good, strong posture, even when you're tired.

Kicking and pulling incorrectly as you swim, holding too much tension in your shoulders as you cycle, and poor running technique will all make your race harder work, and make aches and pains more likely. Study our skills sections thoroughly, and whenever you are out training, go through the perfect form pointers in your mind.

To give some examples, an incorrect head and neck position can lead to tension and straining in the shoulders, upper back and neck in the pool. Breaststroke swimmers whose knees twist as they kick often end up with sore kneecaps, too. Cyclists who pedal without good technique risk knee injury, and runners who twist as they move place added pressure on their knees, hips and back.

Improve your 'core' stability

All the coaches we spoke to agreed that weak core stability is one of the main contributing factors to injury in triathletes. Core stability is the ability to control the midsection of your body through the use of the muscles that surround your torso, connecting to your spine, pelvis and shoulders. Good core stability is important for good posture, and provides the foundation for arm and leg movements.

'If your core muscles are weak, your body compensates by overusing other muscle groups,' says sports physiotherapist Sammy Margo. Follow the core programme on pages 162–3 twice a week.

Don't forget to stretch

Stretching after a training session is often overlooked; this can lead to tighter muscles that are more liable to cramp or tear, which could ruin a training session or race. Stretch your hip flexors, hamstrings and quadriceps after every swim, ride or run (see pages 60–7 for the post-exercise stretch programme).

Triathlon coach and GB competitor Ralph Hydes says that pulling a muscle 'is often associated with exercising cold, without warming up. But if a muscle is going to go, it is a result of a build-up of tension.' Think of your stretching programme as insurance against injury.

What if I do get injured?

It isn't uncommon to sustain an injury, particularly if you're new to triathlon, but many of the most common injuries are simple to treat, and don't have to ruin your racing ambitions. If you do get injured, ask your GP to refer you to a physiotherapist, who will be able to check you over and recommend suitable exercises. Here, we run through the most common tri training injuries and how to aid your recovery.

Kneecap pain
Common in cyclists and runners, this can have many causes. Pain can result from incorrect alignment of the knee as you run or cycle, or overuse. The resulting inflammation makes the knee feel tender, and training painful.

To ease kneecap pain, stretch your knees after exercise. A good way is to bend your knee and hold your heel into your buttock, so you feel a stretch over your kneecap. The Lizard and Pigeon poses (see pages 62 and 65) also work. If your knees still feel sore, soothe with a bag of ice or frozen vegetables.

Swimmer's shoulder
Although swimming injuries are fairly uncommon, a survey of 1200 elite swimmers found that almost three-quarters had experienced shoulder pain at some point. Most physios believe this is due to the

irritation of the shoulder cuff muscles that control rotation, and sometimes also as a result of instability in the shoulder joint.

To ease painful shoulders, increase your warm-up period before a training session, and place a bag of ice or frozen vegetables on your shoulders after training. To avoid future strain, the strengthening exercises recommended in the core programme (see pages 162–3) should help redress any muscle imbalances you may have.

Foot pain
Plantar fasciitis is by far the most common cause of foot pain in runners, and results from inflammation of the tendon that supports the arch of your foot. Common symptoms are heel pain that is worst first thing in the day and at the start of a training session. It is more common in those who either overpronate or supinate (see page 131), and it can be exacerbated by unsupportive footwear and lack of stretching. It often develops after a sudden increase in activity.

To ease foot pain, stretch your feet daily. Sitting in a chair, cross one foot over the opposite knee, and with your hand, bend your toes back towards your shin. Hold for ten seconds, then swap sides. You can also try rolling a tennis ball between the arch of your foot and the floor. Orthotic insoles (see page 132) can help.

The stretches

Stretching is something that is often forgotten by triathletes, a mistake that can lead to injury and discomfort.

It's easy to forget stretching altogether when you're worrying about fitting your training sessions into a busy schedule, but this is a false economy, as an effective stretching programme aids muscle repair, guards against injury, boosts flexibility, and can improve your posture and form.

If you have time, attending a regular yoga class will bring real benefits to your triathlon-training programme. But even if you don't, you can reap the benefits by incorporating these stretches into your warm-down. Yoga teacher Laura Denham-Jones, who has created a yoga class specifically for sports such as long-distance running and triathlon, devised the stretch programme that follows. 'These postures will help to realign your body, releasing pent-up muscle tension, and easing out the "kinks" that are commonly caused by a demanding training programme. Triathletes are particularly prone to tight legs, buttocks, hips, backs and shoulders, so the stretches that follow focus on these areas.'

If you were to do all the postures below after a training session, it should take only 10–15 minutes. But if you are more pressed for time, spend a minimum of 5 minutes doing a selection that work your whole body. Whatever you do, ensure you spend at least 30 seconds in each pose (unless otherwise instructed), as doing so will allow a deeper stretch in your muscles and connective tissue. Breathe deeply throughout to help relax your body and mind.

What you'll need

- An exercise or yoga mat
- Some yoga blocks
  (if you don't have these, books at least 5cm thick can be used)
- A yoga or exercise strap or belt
  (optional)
- A wall

A note on breathing

Ensuring your breath is relaxed and full during the stretch sequence will enable you to get the most from it, as it will help you to hold each stretch comfortably. Most people breathe too quickly and shallowly, which means you don't utilise your full lung capacity. This is particularly true after a race or training session, when you're trying to catch your breath. In yoga it's recommended to breathe in and out through your nose, and breathe in as you prepare for a stretch, breathing out on the effort (whether you're bending, stretching or twisting). You should aim to breathe evenly and deeply throughout: 'If you can't breathe comfortably in a stretch, you shouldn't be doing it – it's a sign you're overstraining,' says Laura Denham-Jones.

Building an awareness of your breath will help your training, too: 'Think of it as an inbuilt heart-rate monitor,' explains Denham-Jones. 'It's a great way to gauge your level of exertion, and you should find breathing deeply, rather than just quickly, when you're working hard helps to energise you.' It's also a good way to distract yourself from how much further or longer you have to go: 'Simply tuning into your breath and listening to its rhythm will have a calming, meditative effect,' she says.

Upper-calf stretch

You can do this stretch after a training run or cycle, too, using a wall or tree for support. It particularly targets the calves and ankles.

1. With your hands at shoulder height, push against a wall, with your right leg slightly bent and your left leg extended behind you.
2. Keep both heels flat on the floor, with both feet facing directly forwards. Lean forwards, pressing into the wall, and feel the stretch in your right calf. Hold for 60 seconds. Take care not to arch your back. Repeat on the other side.

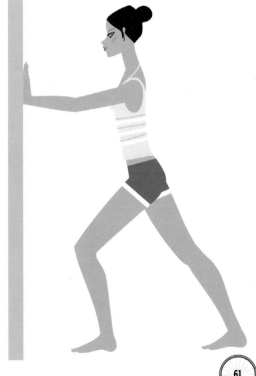

Forward bend against a wall

This provides a good stretch up the back of your legs, especially in the calves and hamstrings. It also helps to relieve tension in your lower back.

1. Stand with your back and bottom touching a wall. Place your feet hip-width apart, pointing forward.
2. Bend forward, reaching down until your fingertips rest on the floor, or as near to the front of your toes as possible. Don't strain or 'bounce' and keep your knees bent, if necessary. Hold for 60 seconds, and as you breathe, ease further down, using the wall for support.

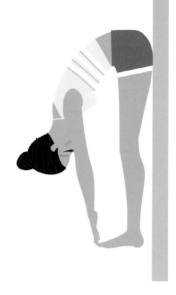

Downward dog

This yoga position is a great way to stretch and relax your hamstrings, calves and back. Initially this position can be tough, particularly if you have tight hamstrings and calves. You may find that you need to bend your knees slightly and keep your heels raised.

1. Start on your hands and knees with your legs hip-width apart, and your arms shoulder-width apart. Your middle fingers should be parallel, pointing forward. Roll your elbows outwards.
2. Breathe in, curling your toes under as if you're about to stand on

your tiptoes. Breathe out and lift your knees, sending your hips up and back.
3. Straighten your legs and push through your arms. The aim is to lengthen your spine while keeping your legs straight. Don't worry if your heels won't reach the ground, or your legs have a slight bend in them.
4. Keep your shoulders down and ensure your weight is evenly distributed between your hands and feet. Hold the position for 60 seconds, breathing in and out through your nose.

Lizard posture

This position is good for your quadriceps, hip flexors and hamstrings. The stretch can feel intense at first, and most people need to use a block or book until they get used to it.

1. From the downward dog position, step your right foot forwards between your hands.
2. Move both hands to the inside of your right foot. Lower your left knee to the floor, so the mat is touching your leg just above your kneecap.

3. Bring your forearms down, either on to the floor if you can, or on a block or book, bending at the elbows. You will feel the front of your left hip and thigh stretching, and the underside of your right thigh and bottom.
4. Stay in position for 8 breaths, then raise your forearms off the floor, straighten your back leg, and step forwards into a standing forward bend.
5. After a few breaths, stand up and repeat with the opposite leg.

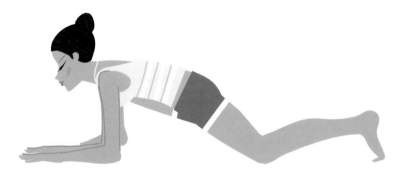

The triangle

This is a sideways bend that stretches your sides and hamstrings.

1. Stand with your feet about one leg-length apart. Turn your right foot out 90° and your left foot in 30°. Your right heel should be in line with the arch of your left foot.

2. Breathe out and bend from your hips, moving your torso sideways towards your right leg. Bring your right hand to your right shin or ankle.

3. Stretch your left arm straight up, feeling the stretch through your ribcage and sides.

4. Look up at your left hand by rotating your ribcage upwards, rather than just turning your neck. Hold for 20–30 seconds, coming up slowly to avoid straining. Throughout the posture, take care to keep your thigh muscles engaged and your kneecaps lifted. Repeat on the other side.

Arm stretch

This stretches the triceps, shoulders, upper back and chest. If you find this difficult at first, use an exercise band or strap to help.

1. Breathe in and stretch your right arm out sideways, parallel to the floor. Turn your arm anti-clockwise until your thumb points behind you and your palm faces the ceiling.
2. Breathe out, and sweep your arm behind you, tucking your forearm into the hollow of your lower back.
3. Roll your shoulders back and work your forearm up your back until almost parallel to your spine.
4. Breathe in, and stretch your left arm straight up in the air. Breathe out, and bend your elbow, reaching down for your right hand. If possible, hook your fingers. If not, hold the stretch where you can, or use a band or strap.
5. Lift your left elbow towards the ceiling and move your right elbow towards the floor. Tuck in your shoulder blades. Hold for 60 seconds. Repeat on the other side.

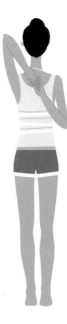

Pigeon stretch

You should feel the stretch in your hips, bottom, and inner and outer thighs.

1. Start on your hands and knees with your legs hip-width apart, and your arms shoulder-width apart.
2. Slide your right knee forward towards your right wrist, and tuck your foot in front of your left hip.

3. Slide your left leg straight out behind you, with the underside of your foot facing the ceiling.
4. Place your hands on the floor and, if you can, walk them forwards on to your elbows or all the way down to bring your forehead to the mat. Rest your body weight over your right leg.
5. Breathe out and hold the position for at least 60 seconds. Repeat on the other side.

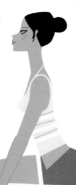

Gluteal stretch

This targets your glutes (buttock muscles), hamstrings and outer thighs.

1. Lie on your back with your knees bent. Take your right leg across your left, so your right ankle rests just above your left knee and your right knee points out to the side.

2. Hold your left thigh, then draw your left leg in towards your chest, so it carries your right leg with it. Keep your right knee turned out to the side, and the back of your hips on the floor, feeling the stretch in your bottom and outer thigh. To intensify the stretch, grasp your left shin, rather than your thigh. Hold for 60 seconds. Repeat on the other side.

The cow face

This stretches the hips, thighs, glutes and iliotibial band (the tendons and muscle fibres that run along the side of your thigh, attaching your glutes and hips to your kneecaps). This stretch is best avoided if you have a knee injury.

1. Start on your hands and knees with your legs hip-width apart, and your arms shoulder-width apart.
2. Cross your left knee behind your right, placing it on the floor. Your feet should be slightly wider than hip-distance apart, with the tops of your feet on the floor and your toes pointing back.
3. Gently lower yourself to sit between your feet. If this is uncomfortable, or you sense any knee pain, sit on a block or book.

4. Rest both hands on your top knee, or if you can, fold your body forwards taking your hands to the floor on either side of you, keeping your bottom on the floor. Hold for 60 seconds. Repeat on the other side.

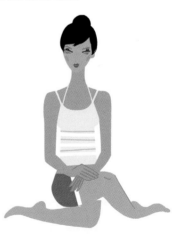

Side twist

This is a good all-over stretch, targeting the shoulders, lower back, outer hips and hamstrings.

1. Lie on your back with your arms stretched out to the sides. Turn your palms to face the ceiling.
2. Bend your knees, and lower them towards your left. Extend your right leg sideways to the left, straightening your left leg, ankle resting on the floor.

3. If you can, hold your right foot with your left hand. If not, use a strap to wrap around your right foot, and hold in your right hand, or simply hold the stretch, keeping your arms spread out.
4. Turn your head to the right, pressing your left shoulder towards the floor. Hold for 60 seconds. Repeat on the other side.

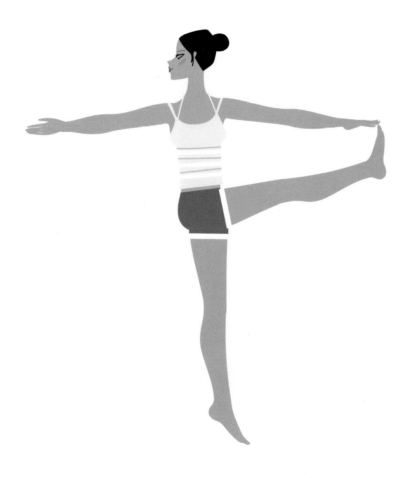

Whether you're looking to lose weight, or simply want to ensure you're getting the best range of nutrients to support your body while you're training, we've got the facts. From calorie counting to supplements, refuelling to superfoods, don't go to the supermarket until you've read this section.

6

what to eat

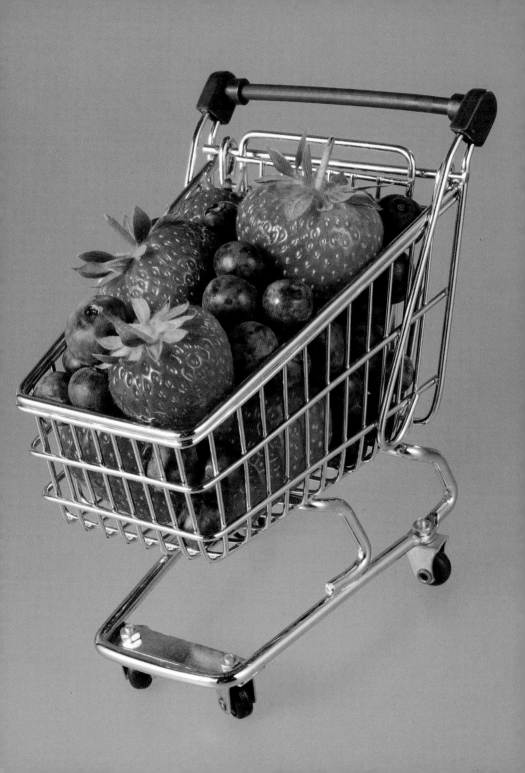

The food rules

You need to eat well when you're training to provide your body with energy and vital nutrients to help support muscle growth and repair.

Breakfast like a king

Even if you struggle to stomach food first thing, the benefits of eating breakfast should make you sit up and take notice. Studies show that dieters who eat breakfast consume fewer calories on average over the day, and are less likely to reach for unhealthy snacks such as biscuits. Breakfast also improves concentration and energy levels, and can play a crucial role in helping towards your five portions of fruit and vegetables a day. Porridge or muesli served with milk and berries, or wholemeal toast with peanut butter, are great breakfast foods for triathletes in training.

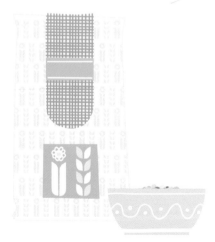

Don't scrimp on calories

'Calorie levels of less than 1000 a day are too few,' says sports dietician Dr Carrie Ruxton. 'If you're doing a lot of training, even 1500 calories a day won't provide enough energy.' If you are hoping to lose weight, Ruxton suggests cutting back on nonessential foods such as alcohol, confectionery and fizzy drinks rather than reducing your calorie intake across the board. 'Fill up on nutritious complex carbs, lean protein and piles of fruit and veg.' As a guideline, a 28-year-old 10 stone woman doing three hours' training per week (as recommended in our Super-Sprint plan, see page 148), should be eating 2133 calories a day to maintain her weight, or 1633 to lose 1lb per week. A 12 stone man of the same age, following the same plan, should be eating 2748 calories a day to maintain his weight, or 2248 to lose 1lb per week.

Consult our guide on page 75 to find out how many calories you should be eating.

Choose protein carefully

Include some quality protein at every meal – good sources include lean red meat, poultry, eggs, oily fish, tofu or lentils. Knowing a lean, free-range chicken breast is preferable to a fatty, heavily processed beef burger isn't rocket science, but the business of making informed protein choices can be more complex. It is worth paying a little extra for an excellent cut of beef tenderloin, for example – you won't notice the lack of fat as the meat will be naturally succulent, whereas cheaper, fattier cuts won't taste as good. Avoid eating large amounts of cheese and cream as they are high in saturated fat and calories.

Think about GI

Knowing the glycemic index (GI) value of foods (the rate at which they release glucose into your system) is useful for anyone training for a triathlon. But although some GI diet books would have you believe that anything with a high rating should be avoided at all times, the rules are different for athletes. High GI foods such as dates, white bread, sweetened breakfast cereals and isotonic drinks can be a great way to replenish energy stores during or immediately after a training session or race. Opting for lower GI carbohydrates (such as rye bread, baked beans and pasta), and including plenty of protein-rich foods and healthy fats as the basis of your diet is the best way to maintain a nutritious balance the rest of the time.

Stay hydrated

Being even a little dehydrated can dramatically impair your training and race performance. Aim to drink 8 glasses of water a day. If you find this difficult, try eating more watery foods such as vegetables and juicy fruits, and increasing your intake of herbal, green or rooibos tea. Triathletes in training need to drink more water than most, as you will lose water in sweat. Always ensure you have a water bottle to hand when you're training – even at the pool. Moderate intakes of caffeinated tea and coffee are fine, and in the short term a cup of coffee before a workout can boost endurance.

Remember variety is key

'It's simple – the more different types of food you consume, the wider variety of nutrients you'll be getting,' says Dr Ralph Rogers, a sports physician and exercise physiologist who specialises in nutrition. Aim to buy one new vegetable a month, and vary the leaves you use as the base for salads. Try root veg such as celeriac, butternut squash and sweet potato. Substitute white or basmati rice with different varieties such as wild or red rice. And as an alternative to pasta, experiment with quinoa, couscous and pearl barley.

Get portion savvy

Whether your aim is to lose, maintain or gain weight, it's important to check how your portion sizes measure up and find out whether you are eating the correct ratio of carbohydrate to protein at each meal.

As a guide, a healthy diet that will give you enough energy to train should be made up from at least 60% complex carbohydrates (including plenty of fruit and veg), 20% protein and 20% fat. A protein portion should be the size of the palm of your hand, and a portion of carbs around the size of a tennis ball. Foods that are very high in fat, such as cheese, should be eaten only as an occasional snack, with a portion being no bigger than a matchbox. Instead, try to include plenty of good fats in your meals, such as those found in nuts, seeds and oily fish.

10 power foods

Bananas

A good source of fibre, bananas are a food with a medium GI value. This means they deliver sustained energy, but give you a natural sugar kick as well. Bananas are rich in potassium, which helps to prevent muscle cramps and regulate the heart beat.

Lean beef

A great source of low-fat protein, good quality beef helps to build lean muscle mass. It is also rich in iron – a nutrient that many active people, particularly women, lack. Lean beef is also packed with B vitamins, which are crucial for energy production.

Lentils

A good source of protein and complex carbohydrate, lentils are filling and nutritious. They are rich in fibre, which helps to keep you feeling full for longer.

Potatoes

Baked potatoes are a healthy source of carbohydrate. Eat the skin to get an extra dose of fibre. Potatoes are richer in potassium than bananas and they're a good source of vitamin C, while sweet potatoes are packed with the antioxidant betacarotene.

Berries and cherries

Rich in antioxidants such as vitamin C, which helps to increase iron absorption, berries and cherries are a great food for trainee triathletes. They also have a natural anti-inflammatory effect that helps muscle repair.

Brown rice

Richer in minerals and fibre than white rice, brown rice is a super refuelling food. If you prefer the taste of white rice, consider this: the processing required to make white rice destroys most of the B vitamins, iron and dietary fibre.

Oats

The health benefits of oats are well documented – they help to lower cholesterol, and keep you feeling full. They're rich in fibre, and a great way to increase your calcium intake if you eat your oat cereal or porridge with milk.

Tofu

A small serving of tofu contains about 40% of the protein, 25% of the calcium, and almost 90% of the iron needed by an adult woman daily.

Oily fish

The essential fats in oily fish such as salmon, mackerel and anchovies are not only beneficial for heart health and circulation, they also help to protect your joints. What's more, eating oily fish with small bones such as sardines provides valuable calcium.

Green leafy veg

All green leafy, cruciferous vegetables, including Brussels sprouts, cabbage, kale and greens, are rich in B vitamins, iron and betacarotene.

Do you need supplements?

The supplement market for amateur and professional athletes is huge. From protein shakes to antioxidant supplements, it's difficult to know whether it's really necessary to supplement your diet or not.

Is food alone enough?

Sports nutritionist Anita Bean says it all depends on your eating habits: 'Eating a perfectly balanced diet is not always easy in practice, particularly if you travel a lot, work shifts or long hours, train at irregular times and eat on the run.' Having said this, Anita points out that 'most athletes eat more healthily, and consume more food overall than the average sedentary person, which automatically means they achieve a higher vitamin and mineral intake.'

The concern comes when you try to restrict your calorie intake in an attempt to lose weight as you train. In studies, active women are often found to be deficient in the important minerals iron, calcium and zinc.

Which supplements are best?

Some vitamin and mineral supplements have been found to boost athletic performance and recovery. These include the antioxidant vitamins C and E and betacarotene. 'It's difficult to get an optimum amount of these nutrients from food alone,' says Bean, 'so a daily multivitamin containing a mixture of antioxidants, as well as B vitamins, and key minerals such as selenium and zinc, makes sense.'

If nothing else, taking a good multivitamin is a wise insurance policy for those weeks when your diet is less than ideal.

What about protein supplements?

Dr Ralph Rogers says that most Western diets contain enough protein (around 20%) for the average triathlete, but the important thing is to consider the quality of that protein.

It can be particularly difficult for vegetarians and vegans to eat enough high-quality protein, in which case, having a protein shake for breakfast can help to make up the deficit. Other beginner triathletes should not need to rely on protein shakes.

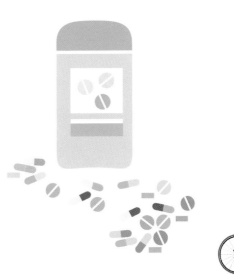

Healthy weight loss

If one of your aims is to lose weight, triathlon training can really help. Even without altering your present diet and calorie intake, the training outlined in the Tri in Ten plans should see you losing up to 1½lb (1kg) per week (that's up to two stone in six months).

If you want to lose more weight, cutting your calorie intake is the answer. You should always keep your calorie intake above 1500 for women and 2000 for men.

This chart shows how many calories you need to cut to reach your weight-loss goal. If you want to lose weight, deduct the number of calories shown below from the calorie count for your weight and activity level opposite.

Weekly weight loss	Cut daily cals by	In 3 months, you'll lose...	In 6 months, you'll lose...	In 1 year, you'll lose...
½lb	250	6½lb	13lb	1st 12lb
1lb	500	13lb	1st 12lb	3st 10lb
1½lb	750	1st 5lb	2st 11lb	5st 8lb
2lb	1000	1st 12lb	3st 10lb	7st 6lb

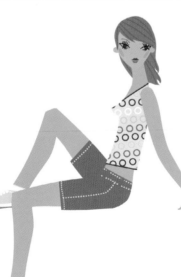

The calorie calculator

Do you want to find out how much you need to eat to ensure you have plenty of energy for your training? Perhaps part of your motivation for triathlon training is weight loss? Either way, working out your personal calorie profile is a useful exercise. The charts on the right show the age- and height-specific calorie requirements of women and men doing different amounts of exercise.

Calories Required to Maintain Weight

ADULT FEMALES: AGE / ACTIVITY LEVELS

WEIGHT	VERY SEDENTARY			MODERATELY SEDENTARY			MODERATELY ACTIVE			VERY ACTIVE		
	<30	30–60	60+	<30	30–60	60+	<30	30–60	60+	<30	30–60	60+
7st 7	1425	1473	1304	1544	1596	1412	1781	1841	1630	2138	2210	1956
8st 0	1481	1504	1338	1605	1629	1450	1852	1880	1673	2222	2256	2008
8st 7	1537	1535	1373	1666	1663	1487	1922	1919	1716	2306	2302	2059
9st 0	1594	1566	1407	1726	1696	1524	1992	1957	1759	2391	2349	2111
9st 7	1650	1596	1442	1787	1729	1562	2062	1996	1802	2475	2395	2163
10st 0	1706	1627	1476	1848	1763	1599	2133	2034	1845	2559	2441	2214
10st 7	1762	1658	1511	1909	1796	1637	2203	2073	1888	2644	2487	2266
11st 0	1819	1689	1545	1970	1830	1674	2273	2111	1931	2728	2534	2318
11st 7	1875	1720	1580	2031	1863	1711	2344	2150	1975	2813	2580	2370
12st 0	1931	1751	1614	2092	1897	1749	2414	2188	2018	2897	2626	2421
12st 7	1987	1781	1648	2153	1930	1786	2484	2227	2061	2981	2672	2473
13st 0	2044	1812	1683	2214	1963	1823	2555	2266	2104	3066	2719	2525
13st 7	2100	1843	1717	2275	1997	1861	2625	2304	2147	3150	2765	2576
14st 0	2156	1874	1752	2336	2030	1898	2695	2343	2190	3234	2811	2628
14st 7	2212	1905	1786	2397	2064	1935	2766	2381	2233	3319	2858	2680
15st 0	2269	1936	1821	2458	2097	1973	2836	2420	2276	3403	2904	2732
15st 7	2325	1967	1855	2519	2130	2010	2906	2458	2319	3488	2950	2783
16st 0	2381	1997	1890	2580	2164	2047	2976	2497	2362	3572	2996	2835

ADULT MALES: AGE / ACTIVITY LEVELS

WEIGHT	VERY SEDENTARY			MODERATELY SEDENTARY			MODERATELY ACTIVE			VERY ACTIVE		
	<30	30–60	60+	<30	30–60	60+	<30	30–60	60+	<30	30–60	60+
9st 0	1856	1827	1502	2010	1979	1627	2320	2284	1878	2784	2741	2254
9st 7	1913	1871	1547	2072	2026	1676	2391	2338	1933	2870	2806	2320
10st 0	1970	1914	1591	2134	2074	1724	2463	2393	1989	2955	2871	2387
10st 7	2027	1958	1636	2196	2121	1772	1534	2447	2045	3041	2937	2454
11st 0	2084	2001	1680	2258	2168	1820	2605	2502	2100	3127	3002	2520
11st 7	2141	2045	1724	2320	2215	1868	2677	2556	2156	3212	3067	2587
12st 0	2199	2088	1769	2382	2262	1916	2748	2611	2211	3298	3133	2654
12st 7	2256	2132	1813	2444	2310	1965	2820	2665	2267	3384	3198	2720
13st 0	2313	2175	1858	2506	2357	2013	2891	2719	2322	3470	3263	2787
13st 7	2370	2219	1902	2568	2404	2061	2963	2774	2378	3555	3329	2854
14st 0	2427	2262	1947	2630	2451	2109	3034	2828	2434	3641	3394	2920
14st 7	2484	2306	1991	2691	2498	2157	3106	2883	2489	3727	3459	2987
15st 0	2542	2350	2036	2753	2545	2205	3177	2937	2545	3813	3525	3054
15st 7	2599	2393	2080	2815	2593	2253	3248	2992	2600	3898	3590	3120
16st 0	2656	2437	2125	2877	2640	2302	3320	3046	2656	3984	3655	3187
16st 7	2713	2480	2169	2939	2687	2350	3391	3100	2711	4070	3721	3254
17st 0	2770	2524	2213	3001	2734	2398	3463	3155	2767	4155	3786	3320
17st 7	2827	2567	2258	3063	2781	2446	3534	3209	2823	4241	3851	3387
18st 0	2884	2611	2302	3125	2828	2494	3606	3264	2878	4327	3917	3454
18st 7	2942	2654	2347	3187	2876	2542	3677	3318	2934	4413	3982	3520
19st 0	2999	2698	2391	3249	2923	2591	3749	3373	2989	4498	4047	3587

Source: Weightloss Resources (www.weightlossresources.co.uk)

Food and drinks on race day

It's crucial to make sure you eat and drink the right amount on race day. Here's our guide.

Before the race

Aim to eat a pre-race meal about two and a half hours before the start of the race. This will give your body the time to digest what you've eaten, and ensure you have plenty of energy. The meal should be carbohydrate-based, but choose a breakfast you are used to eating, so you know it won't irritate your digestive system. The serving size depends on your body weight; don't eat too much, as it will take longer to digest.

The guideline for a woman weighing 60kg (9st 6lb) is:

- Two English muffins or crumpets with 2 tsp honey or jam, or
- 60g (2oz) cereal with a medium-sized banana and milk, or
- Two slices of fruit toast with jam.

A 70kg (11st) man should eat:

- Three English muffins or crumpets with 3 tsp honey or jam, or
- 80g (3oz) cereal with a medium-sized banana and milk, or
- Three slices of fruit toast with jam.

Aim to drink about 600ml (1 pint) of water or fruit juice diluted with water before the start. Allow time to go to the toilet.

If you are competing in an Olympic-distance race or a half-Ironman, eating plenty of carbohydrates ('carb-loading') in the week prior to the race can pay dividends. Do this by increasing the proportion of carbohydrates in your meals in the days leading up to race day. Carb-loading ensures your muscles are loaded with glycogen (the fuel they make from carbohydrate that will give you energy on race day).

Choose unprocessed carbohydratess and wholegrains where possible; wholewheat pasta, wholemeal bread and brown rice are good options.

During a race

It is essential to drink before, during and after a race. You should try to drink 750ml (1¼ pints) for every hour you are racing. If you're competing in a sprint triathlon, you shouldn't need to eat during the race, but for a longer race it's important to do so.

Drinking during a race

Dehydration can dramatically impair performance. Dr Ralph Rogers says that 'even a 2% loss of fluid can significantly hamper energy and endurance levels'. If you feel thirsty, you are already dehydrated.

You won't be able to drink during the swim, but make sure you drink before and afterwards; keep a drink in your transition space.

Keep water or an isotonic drink (which contains a small amount of carbohydrate and sodium to replenish what gets lost through sweat) handy during the cycle and running legs of the race. Try to fix a drinks bottle on your bike so you can sip as you cycle.

Check before the race whether there are any water stations on the race route, and work out how much water you will need; if it's a warm day, you may need two or three bottles of fluid in your transition box. Choose a drinks bottle that you can run with easily, and try to take a few sips every 15 minutes.

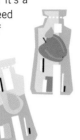

Eating during a race
When it comes to refuelling during longer races, guidelines recommend that triathletes take on 30–60g (1–2oz) of carbohydrate per hour; this has also been found to reduce the risk of sports injury. The easiest way to do this is with sports drinks or carbohydrate energy gel sachets (which contain 30g (1oz) per gel), as eating a flapjack or banana is messy and difficult when you're on the move. Tape the energy gels to your bike frame so you can refuel as you cycle.

As with your breakfast though, it's important not to try anything new on race day. Many athletes have favourite sports drinks – and find that some are easier to stomach than others, so experiment during your training to find one that works for you. Flat cola is still a popular choice for many people, despite the range of sport-specific isotonic drinks on the market. The best time to eat, or take an energy gel,

is during the bike leg of the race or in transition. Some athletes find that energy gels make them feel thirsty, so make sure you drink enough. If you don't like isotonic drinks or gels, try a pack of jelly babies or some dried fruit instead.

After a race
Dr Rogers recommends refuelling by aiming to eat some carbohydrate-rich food within 15 minutes of the race finish to optimise your body's glycogen replenishment. Jam or honey sandwiches and cereal bars are great options. Ensure you rehydrate, too, particularly if you haven't managed to consume the recommended 750ml (1¼ pints) of water per hour during the race. After a tough race, it can actually be difficult to digest a big meal, but it's important to eat something. Pack a snack of your choice in your kit bag, so you can collect it after finishing.

Your race requirements

Super-Sprint/Sprint race
During: 750ml (1¼ pints) water or isotonic drink every hour. Energy gel or small banana if you need it. After: Cereal bar or a large banana.

Olympic distance
During: 750ml (1¼ pints) water or isotonic drink every hour. 30g (1 oz) carbohydrate per hour (up to six energy gels for a three-hour race). After: Jam sandwich or a small bar of dark chocolate.

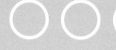

Whether you're a slow and steady breaststroker, or a speedy, competitive crawler, incorporating some key drills into your training will pay dividends. We consulted top coaches to explain how to achieve perfect form in the pool, and got insider info on open-water swimming, too.

7

swimming

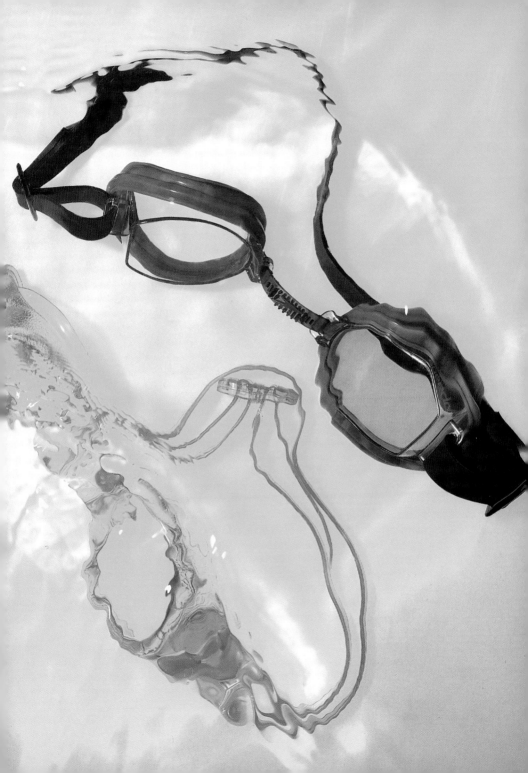

In the swim

Swimming is the part of triathlon that puts most people off, perhaps because most of us stop swim training at school. Many beginner triathletes also panic about open-water swimming, but a few simple pointers should put your mind at rest.

Swimming coach Liz Scott, who specialises in training triathletes, says she has lost count of the number of times she's heard somebody say, 'I can run for miles, but as soon as I get in a pool, I'm exhausted after just one length.'

Many people are apprehensive about swimming thanks to the bad habits they've picked up over the years, which makes their stroke style inefficient and therefore slow, uncomfortable and tiring.

Which stroke to use

It's important to address the notion that worries a number of first-time triathletes – you don't have to swim front crawl in a race (though it is important to note that backstroke and butterfly often aren't allowed). 'Plenty of competitors choose to swim breaststroke, particularly in their first few races,' says Helen Gorman, a swim coach and former GB athlete who now creates Zoggs Swim4Triathlon programmes. 'You should choose whatever stroke you feel most comfortable with.' Timewise, the swim will be the shortest leg of the race, so a slow swim won't affect your overall time to the same extent as a slow cycle or run.

Improving your stroke

It's simple to improve your stroke speed and efficiency when you know how. Making just a few adjustments to your balance, breathing and posture in the water will bring dramatic improvements to your style. 'There are some classic mistakes that almost everyone makes when it comes to crawl,' says Scott. These are:

1. Crossing over, where your hand enters the water diagonally with each stroke, cutting the midline of your body in the water.

2. Leg-dragging, which makes it hard to move through the water quickly.

3. Windmilling with your arms, which wastes energy.

4. Not rotating enough, or rotating too much as you stroke and breathe. Both these mistakes cause drag.

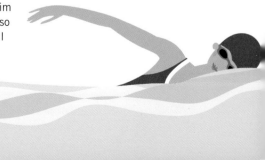

The common breaststroke errors made include:

1. Pulling too wide, which affects the timing of your stroke and prevents you from getting the maximum power from your legs.

2. Swimming with your head above water. This causes neck and back strain, and leads to drag.

Two key points to try

We consulted swim coaches to give us advice on perfecting both crawl and breaststroke technique, and breaking bad habits. What unites the advice for both crawl and breaststroke are two basic principles that enable an efficient stroking technique:

1. Aim to keep your body 'long' and stretched out in the water.

2. Make every stroke count; use as few strokes as possible to travel the distance you are swimming.

Next time you're in the pool, try this test. Look at the strongest swimmers, those who appear the most confident, comfortable and consistently fast. Count their strokes per length, then compare them with a slower, more laboured swimmer. The chances are the faster swimmer is using fewer strokes. This is crucial for good racing technique, as it enables you to conserve energy, and move through the water with the minimum resistance.

Think about your head

The correct head position is important for both crawl and breaststroke, as it has a dramatic impact on the rest of your body. The head is extremely heavy, so it's not surprising that adjusting its position can have a huge impact on the streamlining of your body position in the water. Correct head positioning is key to comfortable breathing, so experiment to find the breathing pattern that works best for you. We have included a drill (see page 89) to help you improve your breathing technique.

Make the most of your swim training

None of the training plans in this book requires vast amounts of pool time. Our sessions will enable you to get the most out of each and every swim, ensuring that you get faster, smoother and more confident with every session. We also promise that you won't become bored (another common swimming complaint) as you'll be focusing on improving different aspects of your technique and fitness each time you enter the water.

'Whatever you do, don't waste your pool time,' cautions Gorman, who designed our swimming sessions. 'Whether you choose to swim breaststroke or crawl, you will benefit from perfecting your technique.' And who knows? Even the most confirmed anti-crawler might change his or her mind after some practice; give it a go – you might surprise yourself!

Perfect form: front crawl

If you want to improve your front crawl, it's worth going back to basics and analysing every aspect of your stroke. Everyone has their weaknesses, so don't be disheartened if some aspects of your stroke are less than perfect.

The first step on the road to improving your swimming form is to know where you're going wrong, and have a mental image of what you should be aiming for as you swim. Swim coach Steven Shaw, who trains triathletes, says that in order to understand good form, 'you have to feel it'. The drills we've devised should help you to iron out any bad swimming habits and develop a stroke that looks like the one illustrated over the next four pages.

A note on body balance

The water should never be lower than the crown of your head (aside from when you breathe). You should lead from the tips of your fingers, and imagine your shoulders and chest are buoys, leaning slightly downwards into the water as you swim (be careful not to hunch). Keep your eyes fixed on the pool floor just ahead of you. If you look up too much, it'll make your legs drop. 'Sometimes imagining you're swimming downhill can be helpful,' says Shaw.

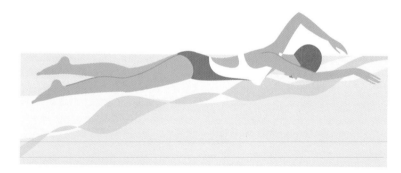

Making an entrance
Your hand should enter the water directly in front of the space between your shoulder and the crown of your head. Many swimmers make the mistake of entering their hand in line with their head, which creates a crossover effect that wastes energy, as it generates side-to-side movement that slows you down. Keep your hand and shoulder relaxed as your hand enters the water. You should initiate a rolling motion as you swim, rotating to the right as you stroke with your right arm, and to the left as you stroke with your left.

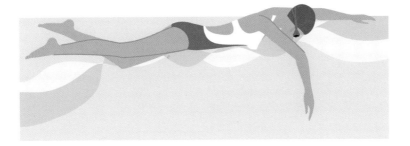

Catch

Resist the temptation to pull back immediately as your hand enters the water. Instead, release your wrist and direct your elbow forwards as if to take hold of the water with your forearm, with your knuckles facing forwards. You may sense a moment of stillness midstroke. Take care not to drop your elbow.

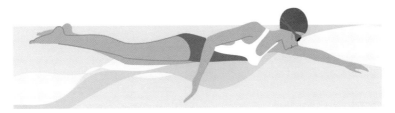

Power pull

As you pull your arm through the water, keep your elbow high. Lift your shoulder blade, and feel your body glide past your 'pulling' arm, which should act as a lever, with your opposite arm in the 'Superman' position. Allow your body to rotate. Your arm should skim your thigh, with your elbow moving in a circular motion.

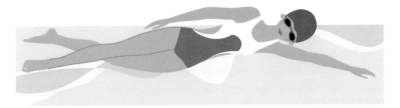

Come up for air

Breathing on both sides will ultimately improve your stroke efficiency, but don't worry if it doesn't come naturally yet. Ensure your head motion is correct as you breathe. You should be breathing out underwater, and breathing in with your head to one side. Don't lift your head too high, as this will cause your legs to drop. As you twist your head to the side, one goggle should remain in the water.

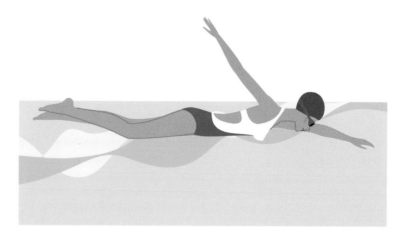

The recovery

Keeping your elbow high, imagine it continuing its circular motion. Start the recovery by lifting your elbow upwards, as if you're pulling your hand out of your jeans hip-pocket. Then swing your arm directly in front of you. Don't overstrain or overreach.

Shoot from the hip

Inexperienced swimmers often have a very inefficient kick, and waste energy with their legs, but a strong triathlete should derive around 20% of their power from their lower body during crawl. Many a coach has urged 'use those hips' – as all too frequently, swimmers kick from the knee instead, which creates drag and wastes energy. Instead, imagine the power of every kick coming from your hips as you rotate them gently, and ensure your feet are no more than hip-width apart. Kick at around two beats to every stroke, with the power of the kick coming from your hips. Think small and supple rather than big, and ensure your feet don't drift.

Think good toes

You should aim for a 'flutter' motion with every kick. One of the easiest ways to make this easier is to improve your toe positioning. Many people make the mistake of swimming with their toes pointing to the bottom of the pool. This acts as a downward anchor and creates drag. Instead, point your toes to the wall behind you, and move your feet gently up and down.

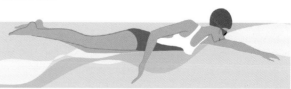

Perfect form: breaststroke

If you have decided you would rather swim breaststroke than crawl, it's equally important to consider your body position and form in the water.

Breaststroke relies more on the lower body than the upper body, and as a result is less suited to triathlon swimming than crawl as your legs will be more tired on the bike. The advantage, though, is that you will be better able to see where you are going, so you'll be less likely to veer off-course in an open-water swim. Many people find regulating their breathing is easier when swimming breaststroke. And if you're looking for body benefits, breaststroke is a great way to firm up your thighs and blitzes more calories than crawl.

But just because you feel more comfortable swimming breaststroke, that doesn't mean you're doing it correctly. In fact, many breaststrokers waste valuable energy and risk injury as a result of poor technique. According to swimming guru Steven Shaw, for every inch your head is lifted (the most common breaststroke mistake), your hips sink two inches, meaning your body is out of line and causing more drag.

Perfect breaststroke, step by step

We asked Helen Gorman to take us through a perfect breaststroke cycle for you to practise in the pool:

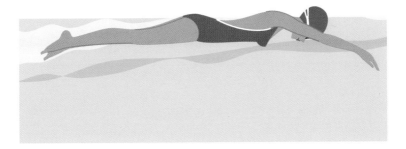

Extension

Angle your arms downwards, imagining your back lengthening and widening. Your eyes should be fixed on the floor with your face submerged in the water. Keep your toes pointed and facing towards the back wall, and focus on feeling long and lean in the water. Breathe out, using your nose and mouth to expel the air into the water.

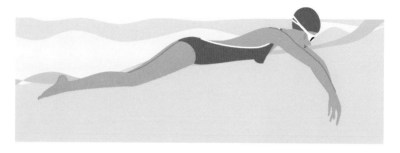

Pull

Release your hips downwards as you open your arms just beyond shoulder width. Your elbows should be bent slightly as your arms push the water behind you. As your head lifts slightly, look ahead. Avoid pulling too wide (this will affect the timing of your stroke so you can't get the full power out of your kick).

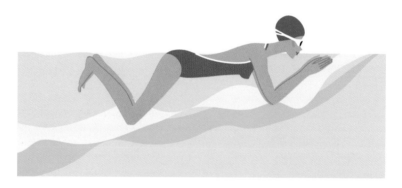

Scoop

Roll your head gently upwards to inhale as you begin to scoop your arms. Open your hands as your pelvis drops further and your feet perform a frog leg motion. Draw your heels towards your bottom as your knees bend.

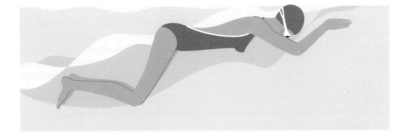

Kick

Thrust your legs back, closing them at the end of the kick and bringing your heels together. This is where you will gain around 80% of the forward propulsion for your stroke. Squeeze your glutes slightly and hold, as you glide forwards. Your head should roll downwards and your arms should extend straight out in front of you. Ensure your stroke is as long as possible by holding the glide for a count of two seconds.

Breaststroke drills

The training drills over the page are designed for crawl. If breaststroke is your preferred option, follow these drills instead during training:

Double kick

As you swim breaststroke, perform two kicks to every pull. Inexperienced swimmers often start the pull part of their stroke too early, which hampers stroke efficiency. Practising this drill will lengthen your stroke by teaching you to keep your arms extended for longer.

Long glide

Swim a length, gliding for a count of three seconds on each stroke. To help you to glide for long enough, count 'one elephant, two elephants, three elephants' slowly. Swim another length, counting down to two seconds, then a length gliding for one second, before returning to your ordinary breaststroke rhythm. See how many strokes it takes you to complete a length and keep track of your count so you can see it improving over time. This will encourage you to develop a longer, more efficient stroke.

Back-breaststroke

Lie on your back in the water, and swim the length of the pool using a breaststroke kicking motion, keeping your arms by your sides. Attempt to touch your bottom with your heels as you draw your legs up, aiming not to break the surface of the water with your knees. This drill helps you to keep your knees close together as you kick. You may need to hold a float to help with buoyancy (hold it with both hands resting on your stomach).

The swim sessions

Here are two different swim sessions designed to maximise your swimming fitness and boost your efficiency in the water. Ideally, aim to complete both each week.

Two swimming training sessions per week is enough for most triathletes. The drill session below is designed for front crawl. If you want to swim breaststroke, see pages 85–7 for the correct technique, and practise the drills outlined there instead.

Most pools are 20–30m long (though there are some 50m pools). Find out the length of your pool before you start, then calculate the number of lengths you will need to swim accordingly.

Session 1: Drills

Practising technique is crucial to ensure you're swimming as efficiently as possible. If you're wasting energy by swimming incorrectly, the chances are you're losing speed. Drill work (focusing on specific elements of your stroke for short periods of time) pays dividends in terms of boosting performance, and it also gives you something to think about as you swim. Remember to warm up first (see pages 56–7). Aim to practise all three drills in rotation, switching drill every 50m

or two lengths. Rest when you need to, but try not to rest for more than 45 seconds each time.

High elbow drill
Why?
This is a useful drill as some swimmers make the mistake of allowing their whole arm to rotate fully in a 'windmill' motion as they swim. Another common mistake is to bend the elbow, but let your arms go too wide. To avoid either of these mistakes, practise swimming with a very exaggerated high elbow position when your arm is both under and out of the water. This will also put your hand into a good position when it enters the water at the start of every pull.

How?
As you swim, keep your elbows bent, imagining you are lifting your arm out of your pocket with each recovery, and aim to enter the water with your hand in line with your shoulder. Don't be tempted to 'cross over', directing each stroke to the opposite side, as this

66 Swimming drills and intervals will help to prevent that aimless, repetitive feeling that churning out endless lengths can cause.**99**
Helen Gorman, swim coach

wastes energy and risks injury. Ensure your hands are always lower than your elbows in the water. If you find it difficult, your shoulder muscles might be tight, so consider doing some shoulder flexibility stretches.

Catch-up
Why?
This encourages you to swim 'long' and with an efficient stroke. As a general rule, top swimmers use far fewer strokes per length than amateurs. This drill encourages you to 'glide' for as long as possible with each stroke. Although you wouldn't swim like this in a race, it helps to train you to develop a longer stroke.

How?
As you swim, keep your nonstroking arm out in front (in a 'Superman' position) until the other arm completes a full stroke cycle. Glide before you start the next stroke. You should touch hands each time. Be sure to pull under the centre line of your body and all the way past your hips so your thumb brushes past your thigh as it recovers out of the water.

Bilateral breathing
Why?
Most swimmers are stronger on one side than on the other. If you are right-handed, your right side will be more powerful. This means people tend to prefer to breathe to one side in particular and their stroke can become unbalanced. In a race you should choose whichever breathing pattern feels the most natural to you, but practising breathing on both sides in training will help

to discipline your breathing and balance your stroke.

How?
Breathe every three or five strokes so you are breathing to one side and then the other. It may feel unnatural at first but as your stroke starts to balance out it will get easier. Make sure you breathe out while your face is under the water and breathe in when you turn your head to breathe.

Session 2: Intervals
Whether you're training to improve your fitness, or you have a race booked and need to get faster, interval training is a great way to get more out of your time in the water.

The aim of an interval session is to be able to swim at race pace or faster over the distance you will be competing in so it won't be a shock to your body on race day. Whatever you do, don't assume that the odd leisurely 400m swim will be enough to prepare you for a sprint race.

The number of lengths you do will depend on race distance and fitness level. Look at the Tri in Ten plans (see page 144) and work out the length interval session you need to do. Interval swimming features in both our Sprint and Olympic plans, though unfit beginners are better suited to drills and recovery swimming. Listen to your body, and take it at your own speed.

If you're preparing for a 400m swim
Week 1: Swim six sets of 50m (or two lengths in many pools).
Weeks 7–10: Build up (as detailed in the Tri in Ten plan) to 10 sets.

Swim at race-pace (effort level 7.5 on a scale of 1–10, or 75% of your MHR). Take a 20–30-second rest between each set.

If your swim on race day is 750m

Week 1: Swim five sets of 100m (or four lengths in many pools).
Weeks 7–10: Build up (as detailed in the Tri in Ten plan) to 10 sets.

Swim at race-pace (effort level 7.5 on a scale of 1–10 or 75% of your MHR). Take a 20-second rest between each set.

If your swim on race day is 1500m

Week 1: Swim five sets of 200m (or eight lengths in many pools).
Weeks 7–10: Build up (as detailed in the Tri in Ten plan) to seven or eight sets (effort level 7.5 on a scale of 1–10 or 75% of your MHR). Take a 20-second rest between each set.

If you're very fit

Follow longer intervals with short bursts of lengths at a higher speed. For example, swim four sets of 200m, with a 30-second rest every 200m (effort level 8 on a scale of 1–10 or 85% of your MHR). Although this will make your swim harder work, the fitness gains are worth it.

Session 3: Recovery

A comfortable slow-paced swim now and then can actually aid recovery during triathlon training, particularly before or after a tough cycle or run. It will also get you used to switching between activities without being too challenging. Swim at a comfortable pace. You should be working at effort level 5 or 6 (50–60% of your MHR).

Session 4: Time trial

If you are following our Sprint or Olympic plan, you will see time trials for each discipline. This is a great way to track your progress, and should be a motivating indicator of your increased fitness and stamina.

Choose a distance that is up to two-thirds of your distance on race day. See the Tri in Ten plan for details. Make sure you note down your time each time you complete the trial. You should be swimming at effort level eight (80% MHR).

Quick tips

Check if you are creating a splash when you swim. The most efficient swimmers glide through the water, so if you are splashing, you are probably wasting energy.

A drop of baby shampoo (not normal shampoo as it stings!) rubbed into the lenses of your goggles will stop them from fogging.

If you cycle to work, try a short swim before you set off; 15 minutes will do. It will help get you used to the swim-cycle transition.

Starting strong

Whatever type of swim you're doing, it's important to think about your start long before race day. Whether you'll be kicking off in a pool, treading water, or diving from a jetty into the water, there are plenty of pointers to help you to go off with a bang.

Pool start

A strong push-off is crucial in a pool start. Begin with one hand on the pool wall, your legs bent and the balls of your feet resting on the wall behind you. Extend your free arm into the water. As you push off, straighten your elbows, pointing both forwards into the water in a tight arrow. If you feel confident to do a butterfly kick, with both legs together, this will propel you effectively. Otherwise, use a few strong flutter kicks to get you going. There will be a timed break (usually 15–30 seconds) between you and the swimmer ahead and behind.

Deep-water start

In open-water races, among others, you might have to swim out to the start point, and tread water until the starting pistol sounds. Practise treading water using the minimal amount of energy.

From this position, you will need a powerful kick to set you off. This is a particularly important start to practise, as if you are used to pushing off from a wall in the pool, starting without one can really throw you. If you know your race has a deep-water start, use it as one of your practice drills in the training programme. One of the simplest techniques is to start with a fast breaststroke kick to get you going, then switch to front crawl. Make sure there is no one directly behind you as you kick back, and beware of people in front potentially kicking you.

Beach start

If you're starting on the beach at the water's edge, once the gun sounds run until the water is knee high, attempting to lift your knees above the water level like a hurdler. Don't drag your legs through the water, which will slow you down. When you get to knee height, dolphin-dive into the water, hands first, keeping your arms in an arrow position over your head. Kick strongly to get you going.

Diving start

Diving starts are fairly unusual in triathlon. When preparing for one, practise your dive during training. Tuck your head in and under, and as you bend over, reach your hands towards your toes. Check that your centre of gravity is as far forward as possible. To dive, swing your arms forward and push off with your legs, keeping your heels together, legs straight, toes pointed and your arms extended overhead. Don't kick too soon on entering the water – your objective is to glide for as long as possible.

Performance-boosting kit

There is a mind-boggling array of training aids and accessories to choose from for swimming. None of these is necessary for the training plans in this book, but if you're keen to perfect your stroke and don't feel the drills are enough, or if you're the type who finds a new piece of kit motivating, it might be worth investing in some added extras. Here is our guide to what's worth splashing out on!

Heart-rate monitor

There are many waterproof heart-rate monitors available now, and they are a great way to help you to gauge the pace of your training and ensure you aren't working too hard in a race. The same monitor can be used for all three disciplines. They are usually worn next to your skin around your chest, and feed back to a device worn on your wrist. Heart-rate monitors can be expensive and are far from essential, but most triathlon trainers agree that they're a valuable training aid. Good brands to look out for include Polar and Garmin.

Kickboard

You may remember standard rectangular foam floats from your school days, but the kickboard, a simple (and cheap) piece of kit, has a multitude of uses. Use it for one-armed drills, to support your arms when you're swimming breaststroke on your back, or during legs-only practice. Kickboards are now available in more technical, streamlined designs, too. Zoggs makes good ones.

Pull-buoy

Many triathletes use these curved floats (pictured below) as a training aid. They're designed to be wedged between the top of your thighs to increase buoyancy, and minimise unnecessary leg movement as you stroke. If you want to isolate your arms and perfect your upper-body movement in the water, a pull-buoy is useful. Using a pull-buoy is also a good way to simulate the extra buoyancy of a wetsuit. It might feel odd at first, but you'll soon get used to it.

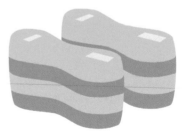

Paddles

Made from flexible plastic, these scooped paddles slot on to the backs of your hands. Enthusiasts say they help to build upper body strength, and develop good form.

Fins

Mini flippers or fins can help to encourage correct ankle and foot movement, and increase propulsion in the water. They also help to develop correct body positioning, as the flutter motion you'll need to use when you're swimming with them will automatically elevate your legs. But if you don't have a problem with foot positioning, these could be a waste of money. Some swim coaches don't recommend using fins because they say you can become overreliant on them.

Nose clip

When swimming, you need to breathe out using your mouth, as well as your nose, to expel the maximum amount of CO_2. Wearing a nose clip is a good way to encourage you to breathe through your mouth if you naturally only use your nose. If you're one of the many swimmers who has a mild chlorine allergy, a nose clip should ease your symptoms.

Mask

These are popular with some triathletes for open-water swimming as they ensure better peripheral vision than goggles. Many people find them more comfortable than conventional goggles, too. Try those made by Aqua Sphere, Zoggs and Speedo.

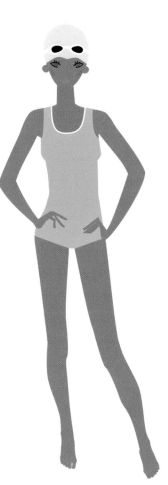

Choosing a wetsuit

A wetsuit is recommended for open-water swimming. Even in warm, summer conditions, your body will lose heat rapidly in open water, so you need a wetsuit to protect your body and maintain your performance during the swim. Wetsuits designed for triathlon tend to be thinner than wetsuits for other sports, and it's crucial to try before you buy.

Should you rent or buy a wetsuit?

We recommend that you rent or borrow a wetsuit for your first race. A wetsuit can be a big expense (expect to pay anything from £150 upwards), so unless you're sure you are going to get a lot of use out of it, opt to rent or borrow one for your first race. You can always buy one later.

When you're buying or renting a wetsuit, the most important thing is to try it on. It's impossible to know how well it will fit, and how freely you can move in it, otherwise. Don't be tempted to buy online unless you have tried the same suit on already in a shop. The size you go for will depend not only on your usual clothing size, but also on the length of your body and legs, your neck size, shoulder width and arm length.

Should I choose a full-body or short wetsuit?

It depends on the conditions you will be training and racing in, and what you feel most comfortable in. The temperature of the water you will be swimming in is the most important consideration. Full-body wetsuits keep you warmer than sleeveless or short-sleeved suits. Wetsuits with long sleeves tend to increase your speed more than sleeveless or short-sleeved suits (the same goes for long legs), as both add buoyancy and reduce drag. However, many people prefer the feel of a short-sleeved or sleeveless suit, saying they lose the feel of the water in a full-body suit.

Check that you can move

It's essential to ensure you can move freely in your wetsuit when you try it on. A wetsuit that restricts your movement will make swimming harder for you, so a pre-purchase check is essential.

Spend some time rotating both your arms fully, and turning your neck as you would breathe in the water, checking that the wetsuit doesn't inhibit your usual stroke pattern. Also, try bending your legs and arching your back as you stretch both hands high above your head.

The thickness of a wetsuit can make a difference to your flexibility and comfort, too. Triathlon wetsuits are generally thinner than the type you use for other watersports; they tend to have thinner zones where you need to move (shoulders, arms and backs of the leg). They also provide plenty of insulation and buoyancy for your chest and thighs. If possible, try on wetsuits when you're wearing what you'll usually be wearing under it when you're training and racing – whether that's a one- or two-piece triathlon suit or just a swimsuit.

Don't be alarmed if the first time you swim in it, it feels strange and tight – you'll soon get used to it.

The good fit checklist

✓ Comfort from crotch to shoulder: This is the most important thing to consider when you're checking the fit. A wetsuit shouldn't feel like it's 'pulling' the length of your torso. It should fit your form, but not be overstretched.

✓ Snug seals: Your wetsuit should keep out as much water as possible. Carrying water will add extra weight and slow you down. Check that the neck, arm and leg seals are tight without being uncomfortable. Ensure you can breathe comfortably.

✓ Ease of exit: On race day, you'll want to get out of your wetsuit as quickly as you can. Wetsuits with zips are the easiest to remove. Also, ensure the cuffs and neck don't make it almost impossible to take off.

✓ Craftsmanship: A wetsuit that is held together by a combination of stitching or glued seams is likely to be a better bet than one that is one or the other, as it will probably last longer. Ask the sales assistant if you aren't sure.

✓ No rub: Are there any seams, zips or seals that feel as if they might chafe? You can use lubricant under your suit to minimise discomfort, but if the wetsuit feels uncomfortable when you're trying it on, imagine how it will feel midway through your swim.

✓ No Velcro: If you have long hair (even if it's tied back), you might choose to avoid Velcro back and neck seals as they can cause tangling.

Open-water swimming

When it comes to open-water swimming, all the experts and triathletes we've spoken to agree on one thing – practice really does make perfect.

Even if you're happy and confident swimming in the pool, the sensations and challenges of open-water swimming are different, particularly when you're swimming in a wetsuit. Wetsuits change the feel of your body in the water. The good news is that they also significantly increase your buoyancy as you swim, and make swimming front crawl easier, as your legs are less likely to sink.

Another open-water challenge is the experience of swimming in a large group of people. You need to be sure of your direction. Learning how to 'sight-swim' is crucial for open-water events, as you can lose a significant amount of time swimming off-course if you aren't careful.

Getting used to a wetsuit
Once you've found a wetsuit that fits, it's important to get used to swimming in it. Sports scientist and swim coach Penny Porter says you should aim to swim in your wetsuit 'at least five times before a race'. New wetsuits can feel restrictive at first, particularly when it comes to arm rotation. This can come as a shock if you aren't used to it, so it's worth 'breaking in' a new suit, or getting used to a hired or borrowed wetsuit.

Wetsuits and breaststroke
As we have already pointed out, wetsuits make swimming front crawl easier, but if you're set on swimming breaststroke, a wetsuit can present more of a challenge. It's even more important to practise swimming breaststroke in a wetsuit, because it will compress your joints, making it harder to kick out. The wetsuit's buoyancy will tend to push your legs towards the surface, increasing the resistance when you're kicking, which makes breaststroke more tiring than usual.

Sight swimming
If you're swimming breaststroke, you're at an advantage when it comes to seeing where you're going in an open-water race.

But if you're swimming crawl, you'll need to practise sight-swimming before race day. Water polo players use a technique called 'spidering'; this is like front crawl with your head out of the water. Although you don't need to swim like this continuously in open water, aim to lift your head above the water every four to six strokes to check that you are on course.

Before you enter the

water, decide on some 'markers' to look for to check you are headed in the right direction. 'It's tempting to keep your head down and follow the swimmer in front,' says Helen Gorman, 'but you run the risk of following them off-course. Practise sighting in the pool if you can.'

Swimming in the pack

If you have done most of your training in a pool, particularly if you choose an empty lane, or schedule your sessions for when the pool is quiet, being in the water with so many other swimmers can come as something of a shock. It is really worth joining a swimming club to get used to the effect of 'drafting', swimming in the wake of the swimmer in front of you. This enables you to move through the water more smoothly.

'Swimming in a club gives you knowledge of where you should position yourself in relation to other swimmers in the pack, to ensure you can see where you're going, and protect yourself from their feet,' says Gorman. 'It'll build your confidence in the water, and will also give you a sense of your pace in relation to other swimmers.'

Expect the unexpected

When you're used to looking at the tiles on a pool floor, some of the sights you may see in open water can make you jump. 'Lots of triathletes freak out on their first open-water swim,' says Porter. 'Prepare yourself mentally – you'll probably see and feel weeds and even the odd fish swim past you. You might spot a rusty, sunken shopping trolley. I had a frightening experience when I was training in a lake once, and saw a diver's mask and bubbles looming through the murky water. I swam as fast as I could back to the shore!' In some races the murkiness of the water means you may not be able to see past your nose, which can be disorienting. The more practice you're able to get before race day, the less likely you are to be fazed.

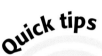

Quick tips

When you get into the water, be prepared for the cold. You will warm up after a few minutes.

If you think the water on race day will be murky, but can't get much open-water practice, swim a few lengths in the pool with your eyes closed.

If you're feeling nervous, hang back and stay wide to avoid the scrum; the swim is the shortest part of the race, so you can catch up if required during the cycle and run.

Whatever your level of cycling proficiency, there's a lot to learn about two-wheel technique. The expert advice on the following pages covers everything from debunking bike jargon to perfecting your form. Plus, find out how to take care of your bike, and ensure it's race ready...

8
cycling

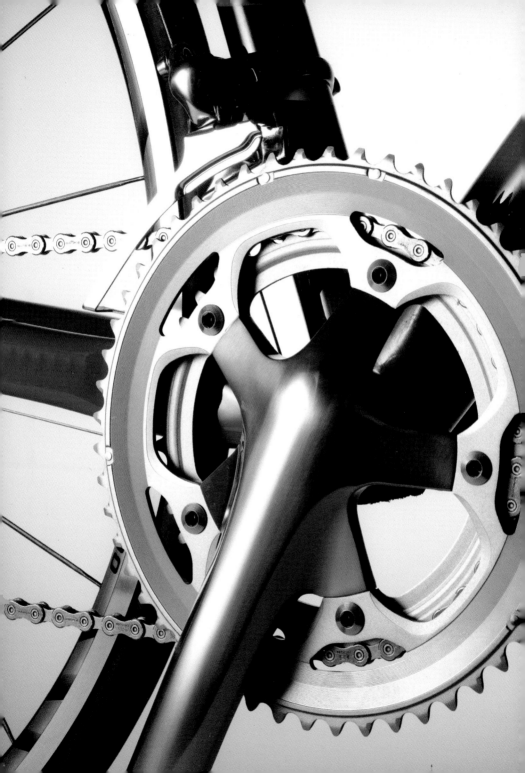

All about the bike

The world of bikes can be a jargon-filled and confusing place! This section will help you to understand the basics about the different types of bike, what you need from your bike for a triathlon, and what to consider if you're going to buy a new one. We have also given you a handy Jargon Buster, which covers some of the basic terms.

The perfect fit

Whether you're buying a new bike or using your current one for a triathlon, the most important thing is to make sure it fits you. Riding a bike that doesn't can result in loss of power and/or injury. For example, if your saddle is too low, you won't get the full power of your leg extension; if it's too high or low, you risk knee, neck and back pain. When buying a new bike, a bike shop will take several body measurements, but here are the basics of bike fit:

- The frame size should be correct for your height. There are specific measurements for this, but a good guide is to straddle your top tube – there should be at least 2.5cm (1in) between your crotch and the tube. If the bike is designed for women or has compact geometry, this method won't work as the top tube slopes, so ask in a bike shop for guidance.

- To find the perfect saddle height, get on your bike, push one pedal down to the 6 o'clock position and place your heel on it. Your leg should be straight, but not locked right out. Now place the ball of your foot on the pedal – your knee should have a slight bend in it.

- Cycle along on your bike – your hips should not be rocking noticeably from side to side as you pedal. If they are, lower the saddle.

- You can adjust the saddle forwards and backwards on most bikes. With your feet on the pedals so the cranks are parallel with the ground, the correct position will put your front knee directly over the pedal axle.

- You should be able to reach your handlebars comfortably. The height is a matter of preference; higher than the saddle tends to be comfiest; lower than the saddle is best for aerodynamic riding position. Any neck or arm pain may be an indication that the handlebars are too low. Many newer bikes can have the handlebar stem height altered or you can have a new handlebar stem attached, so check with your local bike shop.

Types of bike

There are many different types of bike, but the four main ones are: mountain bike, road bike (or racer), hybrid bike and triathlon-specific/time-trial bike. You can do a triathlon on any kind of bike, but some will make life easier than others – for instance, a road bike requires much less effort to ride on roads than a chunky mountain bike.

The basic differences

Mountain bike: Fat tyres with knobbly treads for good grip; thick, sturdy frame; front (and sometimes rear) suspension to absorb bumps; upright riding position; very low gearing for riding up steep gradients. Ideal for off-road adventure but not so good for road cycling.

Road bike: Thin, high-pressure tyres; thinner, lighter frame; drop handlebars to enable aerodynamic riding position. Ideal for going fast on the road, but not so good for comfort.

Hybrid: Tyres that are thinner than a mountain bike's and fatter than a road bike's; upright riding position; some have front suspension; lightweight frame. Ideal for commuting to work or light off-road cycling, but not so good for speedy road cycling.

Triathlon-specific/time-trial: Thin, fast tyres; fitted aerobars with fingertip gear shifters for continuous aerodynamic riding position; steeper seat-tube angle to get the cyclist further forward into optimum racing position and reduce stress on the muscles needed for running. Ideal for cycling aficionados, this is a racing bike for those who are ultra-serious about triathlon cycling.

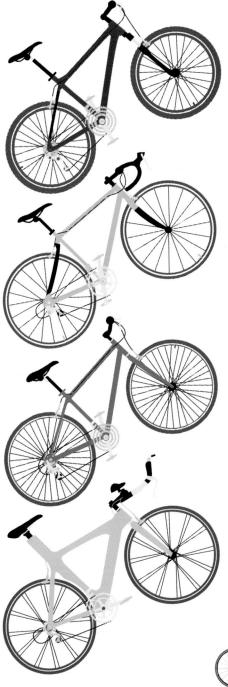

Choosing a new bike

When buying a new bike, ask yourself the following to decide which type is best for you:

- How much do I want to spend?
- What will I be using it for?
- Does it have to be used for more than one reason, such as cycling to work as well as races?

According to *Men's Health* bike test editor Scott Bentley, the ideal bike for a triathlon (aside from a triathlon-specific one for those with a very large budget) is a road bike. 'They're fast, you can adapt them with clip-on aerobars if you want to, and you can use them for everyday cycling,' he explains. 'A hybrid is great if you're a less confident cyclist as it has an upright cycling position and it's more stable and comfortable. A mountain bike is really only for off-road cycling.'

Many brands also offer female-specific bikes, which are designed with a woman's frame and build (longer legs, shorter torso and shorter arms than a man of equivalent height) in mind.

'Budget will be your main deciding factor,' says Bentley. 'The more you pay, the better and lighter the materials become, but you don't need to worry about that sort of thing unless you start to take cycling really seriously.' Between about £350 and £500 will buy you a good first bike. 'Lastly, always test ride a bike before you part with your hard-earned cash – if the bike shop isn't willing to let you do this, walk away.'

The anatomy of a bike

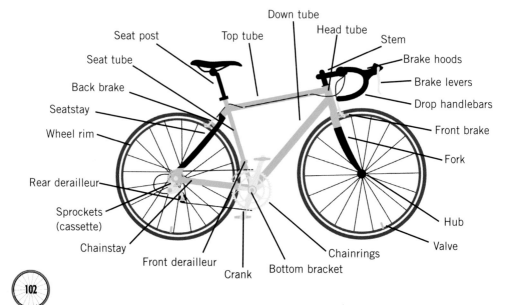

Seat post · Top tube · Down tube · Head tube · Stem · Seat tube · Brake hoods · Back brake · Brake levers · Seatstay · Drop handlebars · Wheel rim · Front brake · Fork · Rear derailleur · Sprockets (cassette) · Hub · Chainstay · Valve · Front derailleur · Chainrings · Crank · Bottom bracket

Jargon buster

Aerobars Horizontal bars that extend forwards from the handlebars of a road or triathlon bike. The rider leans their forearms on them to achieve the ultimate aerodynamic riding position. They can be clipped on or come as an integral part of a triathlon bike.

Clipless pedals Clipless, clip-in or step-in pedals require a special cycling shoe that attaches to a locking mechanism on the pedal. You twist your heel outwards to disengage from the pedal. Clipless refers to not using an external toe clip (see below).

Cycling shoes Cycling shoes have stiff, rigid soles to maximise the power and efficiency of your pedal stroke. They have a cleat on the bottom that locks into the clipless pedal, so you can apply power throughout the pedalling circle.

Toe clips Cages that attach to your existing pedals and hold your foot in the best position for cycling. They don't require a special shoe.

Sprockets The cogs of varying sizes over which your chain runs at the back of the bike.

Cassette The rear set of gears, which is made up of up to 10 sprockets.

Chainrings The cogs over which the chain runs at the front – there will usually be two or three.

Derailleurs or mechs The devices that 'derail' your chain and shift it between sprockets at the back and chainrings at the front.

Cranks The metal arms that attach the pedals to the bottom bracket.

Bottom bracket The axle and bearings that are threaded through the bottom of the frame.

Disc brakes Generally found on mountain or hybrid bikes, they grip a disc on the hub of the wheel and perform better in wet or muddy conditions than traditional brakes, which grip the rim of the wheel.

Brake pads/blocks The rubber pads that grip your wheel rim when you brake.

Inner tube The inflatable tube that sits inside the tyre.

Valves Part of the inner tube, they stick through the rim of the wheels. You attach the pump to them when inflating the tyres.

Shifters/gear levers The levers you use to change gear.

Gears Made up of the chainrings and sprockets and counted by how many of each you have eg three chainrings x eight sprockets = 24 gears.

Hubs The centre part of the wheels.

103

Perfect form: cycling

Being able to ride a bike from A to B is a great start to your triathlon training, but like swimming and running, working on your form and technique will make cycling easier and even more enjoyable.

We asked Glenn Cook, a former GB triathlete with six British titles to his name (www.bodyworkswebsite .co.uk) for advice on perfect form for cycling. Triathlon cycling has a slightly different technique in that you use a higher cadence (see below) than you would in a cycle-only race (time trial). This is because you need to preserve your legs for the run.

There are many ways to improve your cycling form, so it can be helpful to focus on just one or two of them in each training session, and build up to putting them all together. Changing the way you cycle can take a while as habits tend to be ingrained, so keep practising and you'll get there in the end! It will feel great when it all clicks into place.

Get the right body position

'Your body position affects speed,' says Cook. 'The more upright you are, the slower you'll be because your body provides wind resistance, acting like a sail and slowing you down.' This isn't a problem if you're a beginner, but if you want to go faster, it's worth investing in a road bike so that you can adopt a more aerodynamic riding position.

Upper body

If you're riding a bike with an upright riding position, such as a mountain bike or hybrid, keep your elbows in (not stuck out to the sides), have a slight bend in your arm to absorb bumps in the road, and keep your head and neck relaxed. (See fig. A.)

If you have a road bike, ride with your hands on either the brake hoods or the drop handlebars underneath. (See fig. B.) Try to make your upper body as aerodynamic as possible by using the drop handlebars. Keep your forearms parallel to the ground, with your elbows pointing backwards (not sticking out sideways) and at 90°. You can also do this when riding with your hands on the brake hoods.

'Your back should be almost parallel to the ground and flat, rather than rounded,' says Cook. 'However, this isn't possible for everyone because it requires a certain degree of flexibility. Just get it as flat as it can be without feeling uncomfortable.' The same advice applies if your hands are on the aerobars.

For both upright and aerodynamic body positions, you should aim to keep your upper body as still as possible. Any movement is wasted energy.

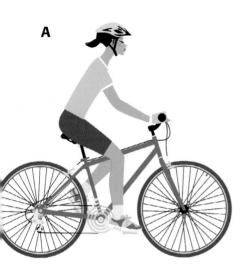

A

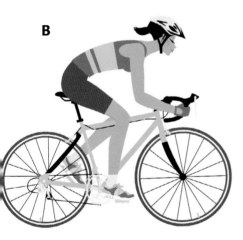

B

A good guide is to keep them inside your elbows. If your saddle height is correct, your hips shouldn't rock from side to side.

Pedal perfectly

Pedalling propels the bike forwards, so you need to make it as powerful as possible. If you don't have toe clips or clipless pedals on your bike, you won't be able to apply power all the way round the pedalling circle because you're not attached to the pedal, but you can certainly make your pedalling count by applying the first two points of the technique described below:

1. As your foot comes over the top of the pedalling circle (12 o'clock), tilt your heel down so you can actively push the pedal forwards and then down (see picture below).

2. As you approach the bottom of the pedalling circle (6 o'clock), level your foot off and then tip your toe slightly forwards to do a movement a bit like scraping mud off your shoe.

3. Use your hamstrings and glutes to lift the pedal round the back of the circle and back to 12 o'clock.

Lower body

Aim to keep your knees as close to the top tube (the horizontal one in between your saddle and handlebar stem) as you can. If you look at professional cyclists, their knees are so far in, they almost look knock-kneed!

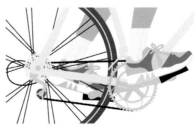

Keep your cadence up

Cycling cadence is the speed at which your pedals turn and it's measured in revolutions per minute (rpm). Each time one foot (say, your right) hits the bottom of the pedal circle is one revolution. A recreational cyclist will cycle at about 60–80rpm and a racing cyclist at 80–120rpm.

Cadence can be maintained by using your gears, choosing one that's easy enough to maintain a high cadence of about 90–5rpm, 'which is what you should be aiming for in triathlon cycling', according to Glenn Cook. 'A high cadence in an easier gear uses less muscular force than a low cadence in a harder gear – basically, it doesn't tire your legs out as much, leaving them with some energy for the run.' A good gauge of whether you're maintaining your cadence is monitoring your heart rate – it should be kept as steady as possible throughout a race, rather than going up and down from bursts of effort.

Use your gears

Using your gears is all about anticipation, so you're in the right gear to maintain your cadence. This means looking ahead and changing gears frequently, rather than, for example, using brute force to push yourself up an incline in a gear you were using for the flat.

You must keep pedalling to change gear. You will mostly use the gears at the rear of your bike, changing between sprockets. A simple guide is that the closer to the wheel the chain is, the easier the gear, or the smaller the sprocket, the harder the gear. If you need a more extreme change of gear, you shift between your chainrings at the front; the bigger the chainring, the harder the gear. The easiest way to get your head round this is to simply ride your bike and click up and down between gears to get a feel for them.

Learn to corner

Don't be scared – cornering may sound like something a rally driver would say, but it's simply how to cycle around corners efficiently! 'In a race, taking corner after corner properly can really help your time by maintaining the best speed,' says Cook.

1. As you approach a corner, start 'feathering' your brakes. This means applying a slight on-and-off pressure on alternate brakes (note that your front brake is more responsive than your rear brake) to moderate your speed before you get to it, rather than trying to jam them on while going round it. You may need to change down a gear as well, especially if it's uphill out of the corner.
2. If the corner is sharp, freewheel round it and lift the pedal on your inside leg up to 1 o'clock to prevent it catching on the road or curb. If you're going fast, push your weight down through your outside leg to keep your weight through the bike.
3. As you exit the corner, get your speed back up by coming out of the saddle for two or three pedal strokes if you need to.

Tame the hills

We all dread them, but here's how to tackle them as painlessly as possible!

Uphill

'The biggest mistake people make with hills is slowing down on the approach,' says Cook. 'If you see a hill coming, anticipate what gear you might need and change at the last possible moment to prevent losing speed. Shift while you still have momentum. It's harder to change gear once you're on the hill because there's too much pressure on the pedals.'

Once you're on the hill, move backwards on the saddle to give yourself more leverage and try to maintain a high cadence by being in a gear easy enough to do so, rather than coming up out of the saddle and forcing yourself up the hill. This is a waste of energy (it uses about 12% more than being in the saddle) and should be reserved for when you really can't go any further without doing so. If and when you do come out of the saddle, allow the bike to rock from side to side but keep your upper body as still as possible.

If you're riding in an aerodynamic position, move your hands to the brake hoods or on top of the bars for riding up hills – this helps to open your chest to make breathing easier.

'If it's a shorter hill, you can attack it by coming out of the saddle as there's no chance for lactic acid to build up in your legs,' says Cook, 'but do this for no more than 15 seconds.'

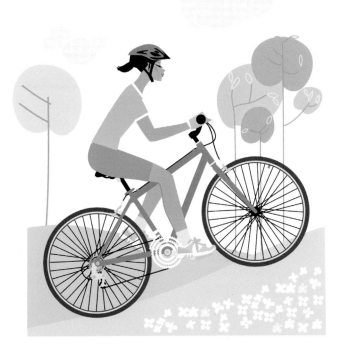

Downhill

'It's worth keeping your legs turning downhill, even if you're going so fast that your gears are doing nothing,' says Cook. 'This keeps your blood moving (it can pool in your legs because your heart is still pumping hard from the climb) and also means you'll know when to start pedalling again as you feel resistance come back into the pedals.'

Go straight

Ideally, you should cycle in a straight line as any side-to-side weaving is a waste of energy and speed. You may find this a particular problem if you're new to road bikes, as they're very responsive to movement. Keep your upper body relaxed and still, and focus on the road a few metres ahead, instead of becoming fixated on the road just in front of your tyres.

Adapt to the weather

Bad weather needn't stop you from training but there are things to be aware of if it's windy or wet. You'll notice that wind will increase resistance and seriously affect your effort levels on the bike (unless it's behind you, in which case you're in luck!). The trick is to adopt as low a profile as possible, so less of your body is resisting the wind. As always, make sure your elbows are pointing backwards and not out to the sides, and your knees are close to the top tube. Be aware that you might experience strong draughts if a large vehicle passes you, so be ready to adjust your balance in case it makes you wobble.

In the rain the performance of your brakes and the traction of your tyres might be affected, so take extra care to moderate your speed early. Avoid the white or yellow lines or drain covers on roads in wet conditions – they can become slippery.

If it's icy you're better off staying at home or doing a gym session. Your tyres won't grip at all on sheet ice, putting you at risk of sliding in front of traffic or coming off the bike.

Quick tips

If you're training in summer, remember to wear suncream of SPF15 or above, especially on your shoulders, neck and arms.

Training rides can be part of everyday cycling, such as cycling to work or to the supermarket.

To stay hydrated on longer rides without having to stop, fit a bottle cage to your bike or wear a water belt to carry drinks in. Or you could invest in a rucksack that contains a pouch of water with a drinking tube that extends over your shoulder.

A note on drafting

Drafting means riding close behind or alongside someone else to reduce your wind resistance and effort. While it's a handy way to conserve energy when cycling in groups, it's against the rules for standard competitors in most triathlons, although elite triathletes are often allowed to draft.

There is an imaginary rectangular box called a 'draft zone' round every cyclist in a triathlon. It measures 7m (23ft) long by 3m (10ft) wide. The box starts at the front edge of the front wheel and stretches 7m (23ft) back from there. You can enter the box of another cyclist to overtake them, but you must be seen to be progressing through it or you will receive a time penalty from the marshals. You should pass through another person's draft zone in no more than 15 seconds. If you can't overtake in this time, you should drop back.

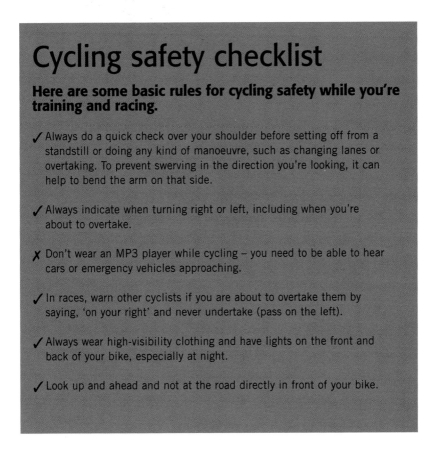

Cycling safety checklist

Here are some basic rules for cycling safety while you're training and racing.

✓ Always do a quick check over your shoulder before setting off from a standstill or doing any kind of manoeuvre, such as changing lanes or overtaking. To prevent swerving in the direction you're looking, it can help to bend the arm on that side.

✓ Always indicate when turning right or left, including when you're about to overtake.

✗ Don't wear an MP3 player while cycling – you need to be able to hear cars or emergency vehicles approaching.

✓ In races, warn other cyclists if you are about to overtake them by saying, 'on your right' and never undertake (pass on the left).

✓ Always wear high-visibility clothing and have lights on the front and back of your bike, especially at night.

✓ Look up and ahead and not at the road directly in front of your bike.

The bike sessions

Now you know what you're supposed to be doing on your bike, here are the training rides that will help you to develop the skills and fitness to do actually do it!

'Triathlon is an endurance event,' says Chris Chamberlin, an exercise physiologist at Royal Holloway, University of London, who specialises in triathlon. 'Varying the types of ride you do helps your body to access all the different energy systems needed for this kind of racing. It will train your muscles to become less vulnerable to fatigue, strengthen your cardiovascular system, and help you to get used to the muscle sensations you will feel on race day.' All these rides will be incorporated into the training plans in the Tri in Ten chapter.

Session 1: Cadence ride
Why?
This training ride will get you used to riding at race pace with a high cadence of 90–5rpm (revolutions per minute), with a dash of interval training mixed in to increase your power. As we've said before, a high cadence is the key to preserving energy in your legs for the run and makes for a less tiring ride overall. Don't worry if you can't get up to or maintain 90rpm on your first few sessions – it's something to aspire to!

How?
Start off by warming up gently for 10 minutes and then start cycling at 90rpm or higher by choosing a gear that's easy enough for you to achieve this. Over time, you'll be able to maintain a high cadence with a harder gear. Your effort level should be about an 8 out of 10 (80% of your MHR), which is what you'll be aiming for in a race.

Every 5 minutes (for Olympic plan), every 7 minutes (Sprint plan) and every 10 minutes (Super-Sprint plan), do a fast sprint of cycling for 30 seconds by going up a few gears and putting all you have into it. Then go back to cycling at 90rpm – the rests in between give your muscles a chance to replenish the glycogen you used for the sprints.

You'll probably find yourself bouncing around on the saddle when you first start cycling at a high cadence. If this happens, ease your speed down a little until you stop bouncing, and then try again. Staying still takes a bit of practice!

Measuring your cadence
You can work out your cadence by timing yourself for 1 minute and counting how many times your right leg hits the bottom of the pedal stroke (or count your strokes for 15 seconds and multiply that by 4). You can also buy computers that attach to your bike and count your pedal strokes (see page 115). Alternatively, strap your stopwatch around your handlebars so you can see the time to count your strokes without lifting your hands off the handlebars.

Session 2: Endurance ride
Why?
Longer bike rides will build up your stamina, an important element of fitness for triathlon cycling as it's the longest leg of the race. Long rides also give you the chance to put your techniques into practice and learn what sort of pace you can keep up for a given distance.

How?
Weekends are a good time for a long ride, especially if there's a pub at the end of it! Get your partner or a group of friends to do it with you to make it more fun. Choose a route that includes a few hills if you can – this will boost your cardiovascular fitness and enables you to practise your gears and technique for cycling up and down them (see page 107).

Aim for an effort level of 6–7 out of 10 (60–70% of your MHR) throughout. Ideally, it should be an uninterrupted ride, so try to avoid busy streets where you'll be stopping and starting for traffic lights and cars. If you can, put your bike in the car or on the train and go to the nearest big park or countryside area.

Session 3: Brick
Why?
A brick session is a bike ride followed by a run and is crucial preparation for a race. The transition from the bike to the run can make your legs feel a bit strange for the first part of the run – some people's legs feel leaden, some feel jelly-like, some just plain tired (see pages 142–143). You use different leg muscles for running than you do for cycling – brick sessions help you to get used to this transfer, so you won't be thrown by the way they respond on race day.

How?
Warm up for 10 minutes. Try to ride at effort level 7 (or 70% of your MHR) throughout and maintain a high cadence. When you finish the ride, hop off your bike and head straight out on to the run. The type of run you do is specified in your plan. If you want to do the whole thing in the park, rather than riding home and running from there, take your bike lock with you so you can lock it up and run from where you leave it. Alternatively, the gym is a good place to try brick sessions as you can swap straight from the stationary bike to the treadmill (for more on training in the gym, see page 113).

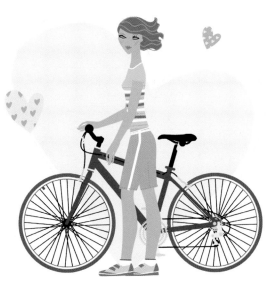

Session 4: Easy ride
Why?
This ride is perfect for beginners or for a recovery ride, as it's conducted at a steady pace and gives you a chance to practise technique without worrying about speed or being out of breath.

How?
Ride at an easy pace of effort level 5–6 out of 10 (50–60% of your MHR).

Session 5: Time trial
Why?
Time trials will be dotted through your Tri in Ten training plan because they're a great way to chart your progress and keep motivated – you should see improvements in your fitness and/or time.

How?
Find a route that's about half your race distance (about 10K if you're doing a 20K race). If you don't know the distance of a route, visit www.gmap-pedometer.com to chart the distance. Try to choose a route that you can ride without stopping   you could go round and round a park if you like – and aim to do it at the same time of day that you'll be racing at, if possible. Do a gentle warm-up for 5 to 10 minutes and then time yourself riding the route. You should be working hard for this ride – about level 8 (80% of your MHR). You can pick out two points along the route to note down as 'splits' – this will tell you how well you are pacing yourself.

One-leg drill

Pedalling with one leg helps perfect your pedalling technique. If you're a beginner, try it on the stationary bike in the gym, rather than on the road. You can incorporate this drill into any of the training rides in this section.

How?
Warm up for about 10 minutes and then, starting with your right leg, pedal with one leg only. Keep your left foot on the pedal but don't let it do any work. Your leg will tire quickly at first but you will soon improve.

Pedal for 30 seconds on your right leg and then swap to your left leg. When you have done two sets of 30 seconds on each leg, ride at an easy pace for 1 minute and then repeat, starting with your right leg. Do 4 repetitions on each leg if you're a beginner and 6 to 10 if you're a more experienced rider.

Concentrate on the technique discussed on page 105 and try to make a smooth pedalling circle with no jerking. Jerking suggests you have a weak point in the circle, so keep practising until you can do it smoothly. Remember to push your pedal forwards over the top of the circle by tilting your heel down, and do the 'wiping the mud off your shoes' movement at the bottom to help pull the pedal upwards.

Take it inside

Cycling in the gym can be a great way to get your training done, especially if it's dark and cold outside, so we've given you a few tips to make the most of your time inside.

Adjust the bike

Before you start, make sure the stationary bike fits you, as it will have been adjusted to suit the rider before you. 'As well as height, make sure the saddle is flat,' says triathlon coach Andrew Potter (www.t3performance. co.uk). 'If the bike has toe clips, ensure the ball of your foot is over the spindle (the bar in the middle of the pedal) and tighten the straps.'

Use the session to focus

You can monitor your performance more accurately inside, as you'll have lots of data displayed in front of you, such as speed, time, distance and heart rate, and no interruption from traffic, so you can really focus on specific techniques such as maintaining a high cadence.

Do a brick session

The gym is a convenient place to do some of the brick sessions in your plan as you can hop off the bike and on to the treadmill. Don't do all of them in the gym, though, as it won't exactly replicate how doing them outside feels.

Go manual

'Controlling your workout manually, instead of choosing a pre-set programme, will hold your attention and make you work harder,' says Potter. 'Try interval training – it's much

easier inside as there are no obstacles to slow you down and you can monitor your speed exactly. You can interval train using bursts of speed or even heart rate; for example, you could do five repetitions where you cycle at 85% of your maximum heart rate (MHR) for 2 minutes, rest until it goes back down to 60%, and then do another 2 minutes, and so on.'

Join a spinning class

Spinning classes are a great way to boost cycling fitness as they provide variety and push you harder than you would push yourself. Many spinning bikes are adjustable and can more closely mimic a natural cycling position compared with typical stationary bikes. The downside is that they display no data, and the pace of a class doesn't replicate a race, which should be a steady, even effort.

A word of warning

Don't be tempted to do all your cycling training in the gym. You need to develop road skills and become familiar with your own bike for race day. Also, the gym doesn't cater for weather conditions and varying road surfaces, so try to brave the elements as much as possible!

Performance-boosting kit

As you do more training and races, you'll probably want to start buying more goodies and gadgets, or upgrade your current ones, to help improve your comfort and performance. Here are some of the things you can splash your cash on.

The clothing
Specific cycling clothing can make training and competing more comfortable, in all weathers.

Cycling shorts and triathlon suits
Usually made from quick-drying, wicking fabric, cycling shorts also contain Lycra for flexibility. They have seamless inner legs to prevent chafing on the saddle and sometimes have a heavily padded crotch for comfort on longer rides. This is useful for training, but not so good for racing as the cushioning can hinder your running.

All-in-one and two-piece triathlon suits (see also page 52) will have some padding in the crotch, but are designed so you can run in them, too. Both cycling shorts and triathlon suits are designed to be worn without underwear. In winter you can wear full-length cycling 'tights' to keep your legs warm.

Cycling jerseys and T-shirts
Made from wicking fabrics, cycling tops are designed to be bright and visible. They often have three-quarter-length zips for ventilation. Most have pockets on the back for storing things like snacks and a spare inner tube. They tend to be long in the back and fitted at the waist to ensure you don't get a draught up your top when you're in racing position.

Base layers
Long-sleeved tops made of wicking fabrics that you wear next to your skin are very useful for keeping you warm during winter training. Wearing several thin layers rather than one thick one is best for breathability and warmth.

The accessories
If you plan to cycle and race regularly, this equipment will help to make your life easier.

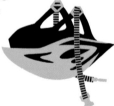

Helmets
The more you pay, the more vents you get to keep your head cool. This also results in a less bulky helmet.

Cycling shoes and clipless pedals
'These are the first bits of expensive kit I'd advise people to get once they're a confident cyclist,' says John Brame of triathlon specialists Tri And Run (www.triandrun.com). 'Gaining power from the upstroke of the

pedal as well as the downstroke can make a real difference to your time.' It takes a bit of practice to get used to them, so don't try them yet if you're new to competitive cycling.

Toe clips
A cheap alternative to clipless pedals, they fix on to to your existing pedals and are good for getting you used to being attached to them, but aren't as effective as the cycling shoes and clipless pedals combination.

Sports glasses
These can be invaluable on a ride as 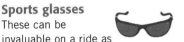 they deflect wind, rain, dust and insects, as well as protecting your eyes from the sun. They wrap round your face for full protection and often have interchangeable lenses for sunny or dull conditions.

Ear warmers
You can buy either a fleecy headband or a thin beanie hat to go under your helmet on cold winter rides.

Bottle cage and bottle
These help in races and on long training rides when you need to carry a drink. The cage fixes on to the seat tube (the one the seat goes into) or the down tube (the part of the frame at a 45° angle to the ground), so you can reach down and pull the bottle out on the go.

Cycling gloves
Many cyclists wear gloves for longer rides as they relieve the pressure on your palms and ensure a good grip. If you're training in winter, thermal gloves are essential.

Overshoes
These are sleeves that go over your cycling shoes to protect them from mud and water in bad conditions.

Aerobars
'Aerobars only really make an impact if you're travelling at speed, so I wouldn't recommend them to a beginner,' says Brame. 'They also make the bike harder to handle and your hands aren't near the brakes. On the other hand, they can be more comfortable for longer races as you're resting on your forearms, instead of supporting your weight with your arms.' Aerobars can be fixed on to most road bikes, but it's important to have them fitted in a cycle or triathlon shop to make sure you're not overstretching.

The gadgets
If you love gadgets, there are plenty to choose from to help you make your training more interesting.

Bike computers
These fix on to the handlebars and the sensors attach to various parts of the bike, depending on what they're measuring. Basic computers tell you speed, distance and time. The more you pay, the more functions you get, such as cadence, and they also become wireless instead of using cables.

Turbo-trainers
These are pieces of equipment on to which you mount your bike to turn it into a stationary trainer – then you can train indoors at home. There are several types and they provide resistance in different ways with varying degrees of noisiness.

Bike TLC

Giving your bike a little TLC now and then will help keep it roadworthy and performing well. If you neglect your bike, you'll end up having to replace parts much sooner.

As well as the basic maintenance described below, it's best to get your bike serviced at least once a year by your local bike shop, depending on how often you ride it. They will replace anything that's worn out and fine-tune your brakes, gears and spokes. Some local authorities or bike shops run courses on bike repair and maintenance, which are worth going to if you want to save the money on easy things like replacing your brake pads.

Store your bike well

Try to keep your bike inside to keep it protected from weather or theft. If you keep your bike outside, make sure it's protected by either a shelter or plastic sheeting, and spray all the parts except the brake pads and wheel rims with WD40 or GT85, which forms a light protective film.

Keep the tyres pumped

Soft tyres make riding much harder work, can damage the wheel rims, and cause the tyre sidewalls to crack. Pump them up every few days and always pump them if you haven't ridden the bike for a while as the tyres lose pressure even when stored. Pump until the tyres feel firm to the touch. The pressure they can be pumped up to will be written on the tyre, but you won't be able to gauge this with a hand pump. For total accuracy, your local bike shop will let you use a pump with a pressure gauge or you can buy one.

Keep the chain oiled and clean

A clean, lubricated chain will last longer than a dirty, dry one. A badly maintained chain will also wear out the chainrings and sprockets faster. Wipe it with a rag and apply fresh lubricant every couple of weeks if you use the bike a lot. Clean it properly every six weeks or so (see below for how to do both these things).

Check your bike regularly

Squeeze your brake levers – they shouldn't feel loose or come too close to the handlebars – your brakes need adjusting if they do. Check the brake pads – there should be plenty of rubber visible and they should be wearing out evenly. Make sure the frame has no cracks or dents. Check that the wheels are spinning freely, inspect the tyres for cuts or things sticking into them (you can often avoid getting a puncture if you remove foreign objects before they've got through to the inner tube), and check the tread isn't too worn.

How to clean your bike

If you're riding your bike regularly, clean it every 6 weeks or so to get rid of the dirt and grime – dirt grinds between the bike's mechanisms and eventually wears them out and affects performance. You can buy lubricants, oils and special brushes from cycle shops.

What you'll need

- Bucket of soapy water
- Cloths/sponges
- Old toothbrushes for bike cleaning
- Brushes
- Degreaser
- Cassette scraper (a tool that fits in between the sprockets), optional
- Old newspaper
- WD40/GT85
- Chain lubricant

1. Wash the frame with a sponge and soapy water, and then dry with a cloth.

2. Wipe the chain with a cloth first to remove bits of dirt.

3. Dip a brush into the degreaser and scrub the sprockets, front and rear derailleurs, chainrings and chain. Make sure you get to all parts of the chain by turning the pedals to move it

round. Leave the degreaser to work for a few minutes. If you have a cassette scraper, use it to scrape out all the dirt in between the sprockets. Finish by rinsing all the parts with soapy water.

4. To clean the wheels, use a separate sponge from the one you've used for the rest of the bike or you might transfer oil on to your tyres or wheel rims. Wash the wheels and brake mechanisms thoroughly with soapy water, especially the area of the wheel rim that the brakes contact. Dirt and grease here can affect your braking.

5. Once the bike is dry, spray WD40/GT85 on to all the parts you degreased apart from the chain. Put newspaper under the bike first to prevent oily stains on the ground. To relubricate the chain, you can use a lighter spray lubricant in summer; in winter a heavier bottled lubricant is best to cope with wet conditions. Hold the spray or bottle over the inside of the chain and turn the pedals while spraying or dripping the lubricant on to the chain.

If in doubt, check it out!

Any squeaks, creaks or rattles mean a part of your bike isn't working properly. Don't just ignore them – they might end up compromising your safety or costing you a fortune in replacement parts, when all they initially needed was a bit of lubrication or the tightening of a bolt. Take it to a bike shop and ask them to diagnose it for you.

How to repair a puncture

There is nothing worse than being out on a long bike ride and getting a puncture (where the inner tube inside the tyre gets a hole and deflates), so it's worth learning how to repair or replace one.

The easiest thing to do is carry a spare inner tube with you and simply replace the punctured one. These fold up small and can be carried in your pocket. You can then repair the punctured inner tube at home if you want to.

What you'll need

- Two tyre levers
- Pump
- Puncture repair kit

1. Remove the wheel from the bike. Most bikes have 'quick-release' brakes to allow the wheels to be taken off, but refer to your bike's manual if you have one, especially for how to get the back wheel off.

2. To remove the inner tube, first make sure it's deflated. Place one tyre lever between the tyre and the wheel rim about 5cm (2in) away from the valve. Pull it through 180° to force the tyre edge over the rim, then hook it to a spoke. Insert a second lever close to it and run it round the rim to remove

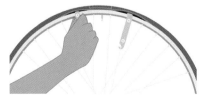

one side of the tyre. Starting from opposite the valve, remove the inner tube and then remove the tyre from the wheel.

3. Inflate the tube with your pump and listen for air escaping to locate the puncture (or submerge it in water and look for bubbles). Deflate the tube, buff the area over the hole with sandpaper and apply a thin layer of adhesive over the hole.

4. Wait a few minutes and then press a repair patch over the adhesive and press on it for about 1 minute.

5. Dust chalk over the patch to make sure no adhesive sticks to the inside of the tyre.

6. Check the tyre by running your hands over it (be careful when doing this in case you come across something sharp), inside and out, to make sure there's nothing still sticking into it that will repuncture the inner tube. Also check the wheel rim for anything sharp.

7. Put one half of the tyre back on. Slightly inflate the inner tube, put the valve into the valve hole first and then tuck the tube back into the tyre, section by section, so it sits on the rim.

8. Push the valve upwards and pull the other half of the tyre back on. Squeeze round the tyre to make sure you haven't trapped the tube between the tyre and rim.

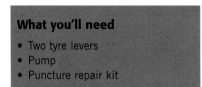

9. Pump the tyre until halfway inflated and check that the tyre isn't popping off the rim anywhere, and then fully inflate it.

10. Put the wheel back on the bike. Test the brakes to make sure they are reconnected properly and you are ready to go!

A little reminder...

Here's a simple checklist to think about while you're cycling.

 Keep your upper body still and relaxed, including your head, neck and jaw.

 Feel the power coming from your legs.

 Breathe deeply and regularly.

 Keep your heart rate steady by maintaining a high cadence.

 Be as narrow (and low if you're on a road bike) as possible to eliminate wind resistance – keep your knees and elbows in.

 Pedal powerfully, making every part of the circle count.

As running is the final leg of a triathlon race, perfecting your technique is essential. Find out how to improve your form and fitness, from varying your training sessions to staying mindful of your posture as you run.

9
running

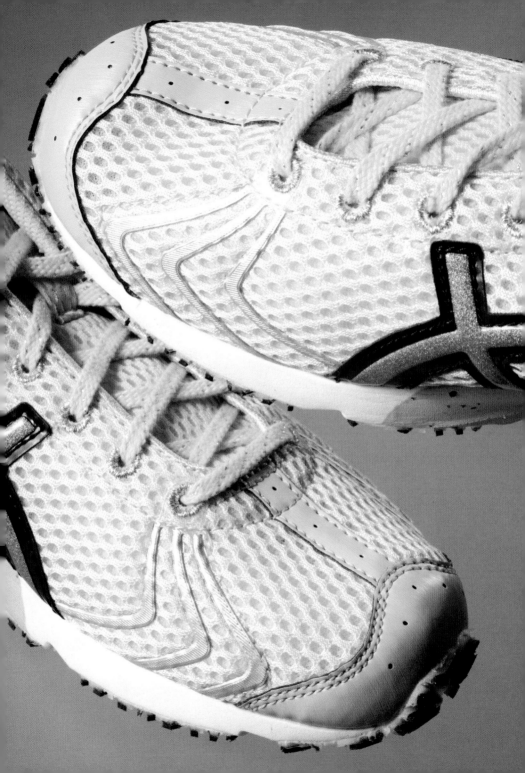

Perfect form: running

Initially, it might seem a bit odd to consider your running 'style'. You may feel that the way you run is as intuitive as your way of walking. However, assessing everything from your posture to the angle at which your trainers hit the ground as you run is really worth while if you want to protect yourself against injury and maximise your speed.

Particularly when you're running for triathlon, it's important to ensure you aren't wasting precious energy or overstraining tired joints and muscles as a result of poor technique. The good news is that by bearing a few simple pointers in mind, you can vastly improve your running efficiency, speed and comfort.

So what does the perfect stride look like? And how can you tell if yours is less than perfect? The pictures on pages 123 and 125, provided by Malcolm Balk, a leading running coach who specialises in advising athletes on posture-perfect running, illustrate classic 'bad' running form, and perfect form.

Where most of us go wrong

'There are a wealth of differently branded "theories" on running form,' says Ralph Hydes, triathlon coach and GB competitor. 'All of them come down to the same principle – upright running, leading with the head, and a balanced foot strike. Most people run on their heels, but the best runners in the world run on their toes.'

Landing on the front part of your foot isn't something you can learn immediately, but by building it into other sessions on an interval basis, you will get used to the feeling, and adjust your stride over time.

Hydes explains that there are three classic running mistakes, all of which can be unlearnt with practice:

1. Overstriding, which places stress on joints.
2. 'Waddling', which is a result of weak glutes and leg muscles. This places strain on the back and hips.
3. Crossing your arms across your body, which wastes energy.

Balk agrees: 'The first step to improving your form is to know what you're aiming for. Then you can try to emulate it in your training sessions.' Even experienced runners can develop bad habits, so no matter what your level of experience, it's worth keeping the principles of good form in mind whenever you run.

Use your ears, too. If your footfall sounds like a 'slap-slap-slap' on the ground, you are 'running heavy', which means you will be placing a lot of strain on your joints. Overstriding can cause you to run heavy, as can hunching over as you run, so check your stride length and posture.

Bad running form

Dropping your head
As your head is heavy, this causes your body to hunch over, which shortens the torso and puts strain on your upper back and neck.

Over-rotating your torso
An exaggerated twisting motion, with the arms pulling across the midline of your body, leads to back strain and reduces forward momentum.

Over-striding your legs
A common mistake when trying to speed up, lengthening your stride increases the impact every time your foot hits the ground. This can lead to injury. Consciously take short, fast steps instead.

Heel hits the ground first
This breaks your stride and causes stress on your joints.

Get it right

When you run with good form, it feels natural, comfortable and powerful. When you're running correctly, you should feel almost as if you are falling forwards, according to Balk. 'This is the natural momentum that powers runners forwards.'

But don't fret too much: 'Although it's useful to think about your posture, it's important not to get too hung up on it,' says Martin Yelling, GB Duathlon champion and coach. 'Focus on settling into a relaxed, comfortable rhythm.'

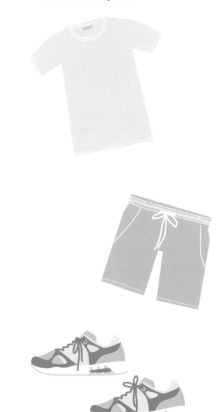

Checklist

If this all feels like too much information, we've devised a simple checklist that you can bear in mind as you run, to act as a gentle reminder in case you notice bad habits creeping back into your running style:

✓ **Run tall**

✓ **Look ahead**

✓ **Relax your shoulders**

✓ **Breathe deeply**

✗ **Don't break your stride**

✓ **Take short, fast steps**

✓ **Keep your elbows bent**

✗ **Don't do the twist**

✓ **Keep the rhythm**

✓ **Listen out for quiet feet**

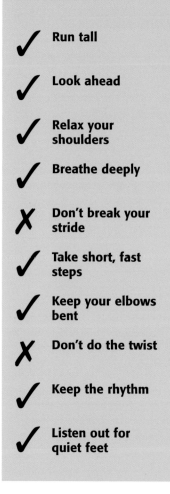

Good running form

Head upright
Aim your head upwards, so it leads the rest of your body. This helps to keep your footfall light, and reduces neck strain. Your eyes should be focused about 10 metres in front of you.

Relax your shoulders
There should be no tension in your neck or shoulder blades. If your shoulders creep upwards as you run, try imagining your head floating upwards, resting at the top of your neck, while your shoulders hang comfortably either side.

Open chest
Keep your shoulders relaxed, and your head high to open your chest. This makes breathing easier, and relaxes the spine. Your breathing should feel unrestricted and easy.

Bend your arms
Keep your elbows bent at 90°. Your arms should swing backwards and forwards in a rhythmic, relaxed motion to power your running stride.

Check your footfall
When your foot hits the ground, you should land on the ball rather than on the heel. This increases forward momentum, and ensures you don't break your stride, which makes your footfall lighter.

Rules of successful runners

There are a few 'rules' that experienced runners and triathletes adhere to from which we can all benefit.

Pace yourself

Although starting out too fast is a mistake that is less likely to happen in a triathlon (as your legs will take a while to adjust to the transition), it's important to stay aware of your pace. When you come off the bike, your legs may feel leaden for a while, and the chances are you'll feel as if you're running very slowly, even if you aren't. Running at a steady pace that you have planned is far better for your morale and stamina than racing off and having to slow down later.

Always stretch

Even experienced runners and triathletes are guilty of forgetting, or not bothering, to stretch sufficiently after a training session. Warming down and stretching are essential to prevent injury and aid muscle recovery after a run. We've devised a series of stretches that are ideally suited to helping triathletes warm down (see pages 60–7). Use the stretches we recommend whenever you've finished a training session.

Stay hydrated

If you're used to running short races such as 5Ks, you may not have run with a water bottle before. Many people find running with water in their hand uncomfortable, but it's important to keep fluid levels topped up, particularly on race day, as by the time you start running, you may have gone some time without a drink. See the guide on page 76 to find out how much fluid you should be taking on.

Mix it up

One of the most common training traps people fall into when it comes to running is to stick to the same route, running an identical 30-minute loop, three times a week. This gets boring, so keep your motivation and interest levels high by devising new routes, and varying the terrain, gradient and scenery. There are great online resources such as www.gmap-pedometer.com and www.nikerunning.com that enable you to measure out new and inspiring routes.

Remember to push yourself

Once your fitness is at a level where you can comfortably keep going for half an hour or more, it's tempting to stick to an easy pace. But the rewards you can reap as a result of running intervals, hills and races will give you a great buzz. There's no better high than standing at the top of a scary-looking hill, knowing you powered your way up it, or beating your personal best time in a 10K. Setting yourself mini challenges all the time will make you feel you are making progress, which is a great confidence booster.

The run sessions

When it comes to running, it's tempting to think you simply need to put in as many miles as possible. But the experts agree that this is not the quickest way to get fitter or faster.

'Varying your running sessions will ensure you speed up, and run more confidently and efficiently. It also makes your workouts more interesting,' says Chris Donald, coach for Purple Patch Running, and a keen triathlete. This applies equally whether you are a novice or a marathon veteran.

Running for triathlon has its own challenges. Running is the final discipline in a triathlon race, so as a result you have to factor in not only the transition (see page 142–3), but also the fact that you will be tired. Martin Yelling explains: 'Many people who enter triathlons with experience of running make the mistake of focusing too much on their other disciplines, and assume their run will be fine because they're used to it. It sounds obvious, but it's far tougher running after a long bike ride. If you usually run a 5K in 25 minutes, expect to add a good 7 minutes on to your time on race day, if not more.'

We have devised the running sessions that follow the advice of the experts we spoke to. Beginners will need only the first two sessions (designed to reap maximum fitness-boosting results in minimum time), but as you progress you may want to integrate the others into your regime.

Session 1: Endurance
Why?
This session is designed to help build up your stamina and keep you going for longer. This is a long, slow run. Your aim should be to enjoy it as much as possible. 'Think of this as a fun run,' advises Chris Donald. 'Look around, and tune into the scenery, noises and sights that surround you as you run.'

How?
If you're unfit, start by jogging at a slow, almost-walking pace. Work up to a walk-run (jog for 3 minutes, walk for 3 minutes). Whatever your fitness level, you should be operating at an exertion level of around 6 out of 10 (or 60% of your MHR (see page 41).

As you get nearer to race day, aim to run for slightly further than the distance you plan to run on race day. Consult our training plans for a guide to how long this session should take you week by week. You won't be running at race pace, but the key thing is to build up stamina so you know you can go the distance – and more.

Session 2: Tempo
Why?
This session is designed to get you accustomed to running at race pace. Bear in mind that this pace won't be as fast as the pace you'd be aiming for

in a straight running race, as you'll be tired from the swim and ride.

How?

This session will change as you get fitter. In your first week, run at your endurance pace, but add a 3-minute burst at race pace in the middle. Your 'race pace' should be at an effort level of around 8 out of 10 (or 80% of your MHR).

As you get fitter, you can do two sets of 3 minutes at race pace. Next time, try two sets of 5 minutes at race pace, and so on, until you're running at race pace for the whole run. You can add a 2-minute slow jog in the middle if you need to.

Session 3: Intervals
Why?

In this session you vary your pace over set distances. It's a great way to improve your speed. Interval training is an excellent calorie burner, and will deliver a serious boost to your aerobic fitness, too.

How?

The best place for interval training is a running track: 'It enables you to measure exactly how far you are going, but is closer to the feel of ordinary road running than running on a treadmill,' says Chris Donald. If you don't have a track near you, a treadmill, or a long, flat stretch of road that you know is a set distance, are other options.

Intervals can vary. You could do six sets of 400m with a 3-minute recovery between each set. Or try 12 short, sharp 200m bursts with 90 seconds' recovery between each set. When

you're running fast, you should be working at an effort level of around 9 out of 10 (or 90% of your MHR).

Session 4: Hill running
Why?

This session is designed to make you stronger. It is different from running on the flat – your core muscles work harder to power you upwards, and running uphill calls for greater cardio fitness and strength. Running guru Jane Wake explains: 'In terms of energy expenditure, running uphill requires significantly more energy than running on the flat.'

Hill runs are particularly beneficial for triathletes because, according to Chris Donald, they're a fantastic way of strengthening your legs. 'Powering up hills will increase the strength of your quads and glutes quickly. You should expect to feel the benefits on your bike, too!'

A note on group running

If you find it tough to motivate yourself to run intervals alone, why not try this variation, which you can do with a few friends. Run in a line, and take it in turns to sprint to the front of the pack in an ever-revolving loop.

'Running in a group is a good way to get used to the experience of pack running if you haven't done many races before,' says Chris Donald, 'and it's a great way to motivate yourself to push your pace, too.'

How?

Try to find two hills near you – one that is short and steep, and another that is long and gradual. Ideally, choose hills that you can run in a loop, with a recovery jog down before you run up again.

The short hill should take you 30 seconds to run up at speed. The long hill should take between 90 seconds and 2 minutes to climb, with a longer recovery loop. You should be working at an effort level 8 or 9 out of 10 (80–90% of your MHR) on your way up, and a leisurely level three or so on your way down.

Be careful that you don't lean forward too much as you run uphill. Pull your abs in, relax your shoulders, and focus on a spot about 3 metres in front of you as you run.

Session 5: The time trial

Why?

This is an occasional test run, designed to boost your motivation and help you to track your improvement. It will show you how much you have managed to improve your race pace.

How?

You will need to pick the same route to run each time you do the trial, to keep things consistent. If possible, try to plan your time trials at the same time as you'll be running on race day. If you really want to push yourself, tack your trial on to the end of a cycling session so you can factor tired legs into the equation.

Choose a route that's shorter than the race you are aiming for, so 3.5K or so if you will be running 5K. Work at level 8 (80% MHR) and use a sports

watch to time yourself on the course. If you want to get even more technical, pick out three or four points on the route where you can glance at your watch to see how your time has improved for different 'splits' (sections) of the race. That way, you will be able to tell how well you're pacing yourself, too!

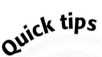

Quick tips

If you're really struggling during a long run, pick off points along the way. Challenge yourself to make it another 50m, then another, rather than fixating on how far you've got to go.

If you're running at night, ensure you wear reflective (or light-coloured) clothing so motorists can see you easily.

Make a conscious effort to engage your abdominal muscles as you run. It'll improve your posture instantly.

Take it inside

When the weather's bad or it's dark outside, training at home or in a gym can be an effective alternative to pounding the pavements. A treadmill will tell you exactly how far, and how fast, you've run, too.

Get on the treadmill

Treadmills offer a forgiving surface, so if you're injured, or feeling a little battered after a tough session, a treadmill run will be gentler on your joints than road running. Treadmills are also useful if you have a tendency to vary your pace as you run, as they enable you to familiarise yourself with what a 10- or 8-minute mile pace feels like.

It's important to be aware that running on the treadmill is easier than running outside. In order to simulate standard running conditions more effectively, it's recommended that you set the treadmill on a gradient of 1–2% – this is roughly equivalent to running on the flat outside. You should also be able to run slightly more quickly on a treadmill than outside, even at a gradient.

Treadmills are great for interval training, as you'll be able to measure exactly how fast you're running, and pace your recovery times, too. Plus, seeing how many calories you're burning is really motivating.

Hill running on the treadmill

If you don't have any decent hills near by, setting different gradients on your treadmill can help you to simulate the action of running uphill. Try running at your endurance pace on the treadmill,

and increasing the gradient every 1 or 2 minutes until you're really pushing yourself. Then decrease the gradient incrementally to allow yourself to recover.

Check your gait

As a treadmill regulates your pace for you, and you don't have the external distractions of dodging pedestrians, runners and traffic, or watching where you're going, a treadmill run is a good opportunity to focus on your running gait. Remind yourself of the perfect form checklist on page 124, and tick off each point in your mind as you run.

A word of warning

No matter how tempting, resist the urge to do all your running training on a treadmill. Although treadmills are useful, they aren't a substitute for natural running. You need to get accustomed to running on different surfaces, particularly if the run on race day is off-road. There is no guarantee the weather will be glorious on race day either, so having some experience of running be it rainy, sunny, windy or stuffy will help you feel better prepared for the main event.

Performance-boosting kit

Here are the key items that will help to make running more comfortable and enhance your enjoyment of race day. Footwear is crucial, and there's a huge range of kit to choose from as well.

Choosing the right trainers

The single most important piece of kit after your bike is a pair of trainers. Finding the right running shoe can make a big difference to your comfort and performance. A shoe that's suited to your gait and foot shape can help to correct an uneven foot strike, preventing injury in the long term.

This is one piece of kit that it's really worth investing in. You need plenty of support and cushioning, and if you're one of many runners who overpronate as they run (your feet twist inwards as they roll over the ground), corrective anti-pronation footwear can help to correct the problem.

The foot-strike test

Try this test yourself to assess your foot strike. Wet your foot, then step on to a surface where you can see your footprint (such as a sheet of cardboard, or dark floor tile).

If your footprint looks...	You probably have a	The trainers you need are
Normal	Neutral foot strike. Your foot hits the ground in a balanced way, without rolling inwards or outwards too much.	Stability, cushioned or 'neutral' shoes. These offer the support you need without disturbing foot strike.
Flat	Overpronating foot strike, like most runners. This means your foot rolls inwards too much as it rolls over the ground.	Motion-control shoes, which offer extra support on the inner side of your foot, correcting the twisting motion of your foot.
High-arched	Supinating foot strike. This means your foot lands on the outer side of your heel and doesn't roll inwards enough before you push off.	Cushioned shoes. You may also require a corrective orthotic insole (available in running specialist shops, and from podiatrists).

Although this test is useful, it's worth asking the staff in a specialist running shop to watch you run in different shoes. Many shops now offer a free 'gait assessment' service, in which they will film you running on a treadmill, and slow the film down to analyse your foot strike in detail.

Getting the fit right

Features to look out for when buying new trainers are good ventilation, plenty of cushioning, and a snug (but not too tight) fit. Be aware that you will probably need running shoes half a size to a size bigger than your usual foot size, and sizing varies enormously from manufacturer to manufacturer. Go with what feels right when you try it on.

Triathlon trainers

Some manufacturers make triathlon-specific running shoes. These are light, may have elastic laces, and may contain a sock-liner. They are more suited to races than regular training, so are not required for most triathletes. Alternatively, many triathletes choose to replace the laces in their trainers with elastic laces. This helps to make transition easier and quicker. You can find them in specialist triathlon and running shops.

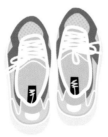

Orthotic soles

Designed to insert into your trainers to correct your gait, orthotics are moulded soles made from synthetic materials. They are tailored to your feet, so they can be more effective at correcting overpronation or supination than specialist trainers alone. Many runners swear by them. 'Up to two-thirds of runners could benefit from using orthotics,' says podiatrist Emma Supple. However, they are only essential for very few runners. If you've sustained a running injury that physiotherapy hasn't been able to correct, though, a visit to a podiatrist could be worth while.

Sports bra

For female triathletes, a good-quality supportive sports bra is as crucial as the shoes that you run in. Wearing an unsupportive bra can lead to the stretching of the ligaments that support your breasts. Once these have stretched, there is no way of restoring their elasticity, so the importance of ensuring your breasts are supported can't be overstated.

Experiment with fit and style, looking for a bra with wide straps that help to keep your chest supported, even if you jump up and down. Triathletes with smaller busts may find that a vest with an inbuilt bra offers enough support. Most triathlon suits will give enough support for race day. If you have a larger chest, consider wearing a sports bra underneath your tri suit or vest. Ensure you replace your bra often (every six months if you wear it regularly) as it will stretch over time.

Socks

The main aim of a running sock is to prevent blisters. Different triathletes have different preferences on the sock front, so experiment with the range available, from dual-layer socks to compression socks (which are said to boost circulation).

The most important factor is to check that they dry quickly. On race day you may be pulling them onto wet feet, and you'll be sweating as you ride and run, so ensure you choose a pair that can dry quickly and won't rub.

Shorts and a top

In summer a good pair of shorts that allow you to move freely and a vest or T-shirt made from sweat-wicking material are all you need. In winter, if you're running outdoors, a pair of good-quality running tights and a breathable windproof jacket should keep you warm and comfortable. For racing you can either wear a triathlon suit or slip a pair of shorts and a top over your swimsuit. In the latter case, make sure the kit you choose doesn't restrict your movement in any way.

Sunglasses

We mentioned these in the cycling section. They can be really handy on sunny training days (and on race day itself). They'll stop any grit, dust or insects flying into your eyes, reduce glare and protect your eyes from the sun. Choose sport-specific wraparound shades that won't slip off when you move or sweat.

Water belt

If you don't like running with water in your hand, another option is a waist-belt with space for a water bottle. Check that you are comfortable running with it before race day, though, as belts can feel awkward if you aren't used to them.

Sports watch and heart-rate monitor

A decent sports watch is handy for training, particularly if it allows you to measure 'split' times if you are doing a time trial or interval training (see page 128). A heart-rate monitor is an excellent way to check your exertion levels during a training run.

MP3 player

When you're training, a good playlist on your MP3 player can give you the motivation boost you need. A lot of running kit now comes with handy pockets where you can conceal your MP3, and although running purists scoff at those who run with a soundtrack, we say if it puts a spring in your step, why not?

One word of warning, though. Make sure you don't vary your stride too much to the beat of the music – watch out for overstriding, or slapping your feet down too hard and never wear it when you're racing!

If you're new to tri, transition can be daunting. But with a little practice and forward thinking, there's no need to worry. We grilled the experts for our step-by-step guide on how to execute perfect transitions. From removing your wetsuit at high speed to beating the jelly-leg sensation you'll feel in the run, we've got it covered…

10

transition

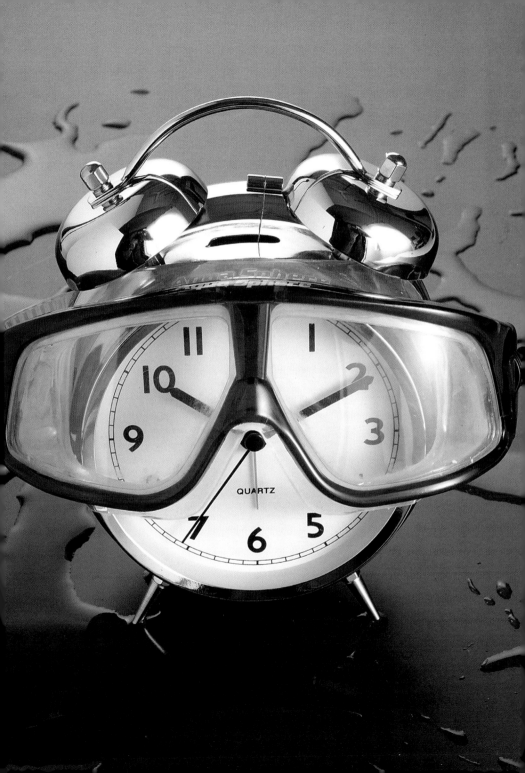

What is transition?

For people new to triathlon, transition can be the scary, unknown element of the race. Some professionals call it the 'fourth discipline' because races can be won and lost in the transition area, where every second counts for an elite athlete.

Transition is the period of the race when you're moving from one discipline to the next. There's no reason why, with practice, a novice can't be as quick as an elite athlete in transition, according to Jack Maitland, a triathlon coach and ex-GB competitor (www.thetriathloncoach.com). Transition is the only place in the race where fitness doesn't matter at all!

The two transition periods
The first transition (T1) is from the swim to the bike. The second transition (T2) is from the bike to the run. Each transition gives you the chance to change into the right kit for each discipline, so in T1 you will peel off your wetsuit, put on your cycling gear, and collect your bike and helmet. In T2 you will drop off your bike and change any clothing you need to, such as cycling shoes to running trainers.

The transition area
This is the space set aside to hold every competitor's bike and kit. Depending on the size of the race, this can vary from a tennis court to a fenced-off zone that can hold thousands of bikes! You will have an allocated slot somewhere in this area and this is where you will return to during the race.

Transition areas have exits and entrances. You will come in from the swim and find your bike and helmet, then exit somewhere else with your bike. You will usually come back in through the same zone when you return from the cycle and will then run out of another exit.

Stay calm!
The key to a successful transition is preparation (see opposite) and staying calm. You know what it's like when you're trying to get dressed in a hurry and it ends up taking you longer because you're flustered and clumsy? The same applies in transition. We've devoted separate sections in this book to each transition to tell you exactly what to do, so you'll have nothing to worry about come race day. Just relax and enjoy!

It's all in the preparation

In the months before race day

If you're worried about transition, give it a go at home! 'I've simulated the whole thing in the garden,' says Graham Walton, GB quadrathlon champion in 2004. 'I've even got my friends round to race me at it!' To go the whole hog, get into the shower in your swimsuit or wetsuit and run to where your stuff is laid out in the garden (see the illustration on page 138 for what to put where). You can practise peeling off a wet wetsuit at speed (see page 140) and go through the entire transition. 'Slow, precise movements are best – if you start panicking, you'll end up with a slower transition,' says Walton.

On the day

Before you leave for the race, go through the race day checklist at the back of this book – it's easy to get caught up in all the little things you have to take and then forget the most obvious (and important) ones such as your helmet or wetsuit.

Before the race

When you arrive at the venue, you'll need to register and pick up your race numbers if not already sent to you. Most race organisers will provide race number stickers to go on your bike and helmet. There will be instructions to tell you what to put where – they help identify you for timing, race photos and security when you're taking your bike out of the transition area after the race. You may be given a coloured swimming cap to indicate your race.

You may also have your number written on your body with marker pen to help identify you as you leave the swim. Pin your race number to your T-shirt ready to put on during T1, or attach it to a number belt (an inexpensive belt that allows you to clip your number around your waist).

Make sure you arrive in the transition area with plenty of time, so you don't feel rushed. Take your time to familiarise yourself with it. 'If you can, walk through your entire transition, including right down to the water, to familiarise yourself with the entrances and exits,' advises elite triathlete Henny Freeman. 'Also, try to watch a wave of swimmers set off so you can see what the starting procedure is.'

In many races you won't be allowed into the transition area to set up your bike and kit until a certain time before you start. For example, if you arrive at 8am and your race doesn't start until 10am, you may have to wait until 9am. This is to allow all the competitors to get in easily, without crowding.

Setting up

Once you're in the transition area, find your slot, which usually corresponds with your race number or age group. Take your time to set everything up. First, put your bike into an easy gear for a quick getaway. Then 'rack' it; hang it over the racking bar by the saddle, with the front wheel facing towards you.

Lay down a towel and set out your kit on it. 'Keep it as simple as possible,' says Freeman. 'The fewer things you have to put on, the less stressed you will get and the quicker you'll be out.'

Put the kit you need for T1 at the front of your towel and for T2 at the back. Make everything ready to use – lay your helmet upside down with the straps open; open your shoes so they're easy to slip on (unless you're using handy elastic laces, which eliminate the need for tying up your shoes in transition); lay your socks (if using) on top of the shoes, lay out your number belt open, undo the lid of your suncream and so on.

Now stand back and do a quick mental run-through of your transition to make sure everything you need is there. Then, and this is very important, take a look around you and note where your stuff is. The rows of bikes may be alphabetical, so remember your letter, or note visual markers such as being level with the first-aid tent. There's nothing worse than coming into transition and searching for your bike among hundreds of others. Don't forget that other bikes will move so don't use these as a visual clue.

If you're not already wearing what you're going to swim in, go and get changed. Put your timing chip around your ankle (under your wetsuit if wearing one) and if you're going to wear long-acting suncream or anti-chafe cream, apply this now. Head towards the swim start with your goggles and swimming cap.

And you're off!

Quick tips

Choose a colourful towel to lay out in transition to help you to spot your kit when you come into transition.

Lay everything out to one side of your bike only, to avoid having to duck back and forth around it.

You can wear your number belt underneath your wetsuit on an open-water swim, which will save you putting it on in transition.

Opposite: This illustration is just a guideline – do whatever works best for you and add or subtract items to make yourself comfortable.

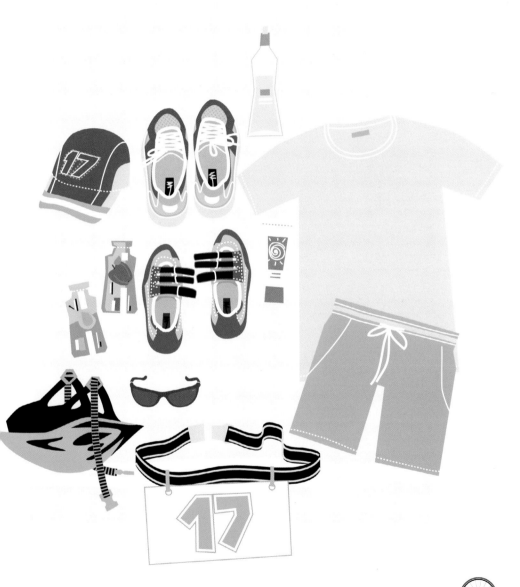

T1: Swim to bike

This is your longest transition as it's setting you up for the rest of the race. Practising beforehand is a good plan; as well as aiming for a fast transition, you want to make sure your kit is put on properly for a comfortable ride and run.

Practise, practise, practise!

'Rehearsing transitions beforehand is a great idea because it's zero physical effort for lots of time gain – you can knock minutes off your total race time,' says triathlon coach Jack Maitland, whose advice has helped many elite athletes to achieve lightning-fast transitions. Here are his top tips for the perfect transition:

Never try anything new in a race!

This is the most important tip we can give you. Suddenly deciding that you want to run without socks or break in a new pair of trainers will only end in disaster.

How to get out of your wetsuit fast

If you're doing an open-water swim, it's essential to know how to get out of your wetsuit with the minimum amount of bother:

1. As you exit the water, immediately reach round behind you, grab the cord attached to your zip and pull it down.
2. Wetsuits come off more easily when they have water inside them, so as you're running towards the transition area, take it down over your shoulders, pull your arms out and peel it down to your waist.
3. When you arrive in front of your kit, use your hands to wrench the wetsuit down to below your knees in one good pull.
4. Tread on the wetsuit and use your feet to pull it off your ankles. This frees up your hands to start putting on your bike gear, such as helmet and sunglasses.

Getting your kit on

What you put on in T1 depends on what you've worn for the swim. If you're a beginner, you may have swum in a swimming costume, so will need to put on shorts and T-shirt. Don't strip naked – you will be disqualified! If it's cold, you may want to add a breathable, lightweight jacket. Don't worry too much about how wet you are – you will soon dry off on the cycle.

As soon as you've put your helmet on, do it up. You will be given a time penalty if you take your bike off the rack with an unfastened helmet.

Put on your shoes. Whether you wear socks or not is personal preference. Putting a little talc in your shoes can make them easier to slip on, as do the elastic laces we mentioned earlier (they could be the best £3.99 you'll ever spend!).

If you're carrying energy gels, bars or snacks with you on the bike, tuck them into your back pockets if you have them (if not, they should already be taped to the bike).

Put on your number belt. Some races specify that your number should be visible from the back on the bike and from the front on the run, so put it on the right way round.

If you're wearing cycling shoes and have practised this in training, you can have the shoes already clipped into the pedals and put your feet into the shoes once you've started cycling (more on this later), but this is really only for more experienced racers.

Setting off

When you're ready, lift your bike off the bar and start running towards the cycle exit. Don't get on your bike – you're not allowed to mount your bike until you reach the mount line, which is usually just outside the cycle exit.

A top tip is to run alongside your bike, pushing it by the saddle, not the handlebars. It will steer itself and you'll be able to run more easily. Practise this before race day, however.

As you approach the mount line, prepare to get on your bike by moving your hands onto the handlebars. Once both wheels are

over the mount line, beginners will find it easier to simply stop and hop on, but if you're more experienced you can get onto your bike without stopping. You do this by placing your hands on the centre of the handlebars, springing off your outside foot, swinging your inside leg over the back of the bike and landing on the saddle just to the side of your crotch, on the fleshy part of your thigh. Practise this at home wearing trainers first, and then in bare feet when you've mastered it. The key is not to jump too high.

Putting your cycling shoes on

It's worth learning the technique of putting your feet in on the go, instead of running through transition wearing cycling shoes, which can be tricky!

Place your feet on top of your cycling shoes as you pedal away. You don't need to hurry to get your feet into the shoes, unless there's a big hill out of transition. Wait until you're into a rhythm and then pick up a little speed as you'll need to freewheel. Lean down and use your hand to help ease your feet in and do up the straps. Pedal again to maintain speed and then reach down and do the other foot – again, there's no hurry.

T2: Bike to run

This transition should be quicker than T1 as there's less to do! Here are Jack Maitland's T2 tips.

Approaching T2

You may have heard that spinning your legs really fast in an easy gear towards the end of the bike leg can help reduce the lactic acid in your legs in preparation for the run. While this can work and is worth trying, a far more important way of making sure your legs are ready for the run is maintaining a high cadence throughout the bike leg.

As explained on page 106, a low cadence (60rpm to 70rpm) and harder gears requires greater muscular force and tires your legs out. A high cadence (90rpm to 95rpm) with easier gears means there will be energy left in your legs for the run.

As you approach the dismount line at the end of the bike leg, you'll need to start slowing down so that you don't shoot over it and get a time penalty. If you're wearing cycling shoes (and, again, if you have practised this in training), you should take your feet out of the shoes at a suitable point in the last section of the ride. If the last section is straightforward, you can leave this as late as the final 50m. As you approach the dismount line, slow down to running speed and bring your hands to the top of your bars then swing one leg over the saddle. Lean the bike slightly away from your body to create some space and bring that leg through the gap so you can step off just before the dismount line without falling over your feet.

Practise this with training shoes on initially, then progress to bare feet when you are competent at the basic technique. If you're a beginner or would rather not try this, simply bring the bike to a halt and get off.

As soon as you have dismounted, bring your hand down to your saddle as before and run back to your allotted space. You must rack your bike back in its original place – don't be tempted to just rack it anywhere to save time or you will get a time penalty.

Wheel it in forwards and as soon as the bike is back in place (and not a second before or you will get a time penalty), unclip your helmet.

Pull on your running shoes (if you're not already wearing them) and anything else you wear for the run, such as a cap, and turn your number belt round so it's facing the front. If you need more fluids, have a quick drink (there should be water stations on the run if it's a longer race, such as Olympic distance). Apply more suncream if you feel you need it and if you need more energy gels or bars for the run, restock your pockets – then off you go!

How to run out of transition

The first bit of the run is the famous leaden/jelly-leg time, as your muscles adjust from cycling to running. This sensation will wear off after a few minutes, so do try to run through it if you can and rest assured that every other person in the race is experiencing the same thing! Try to focus on two key things as you run out of transition:

- Run as upright as possible, with your hips thrusting forwards – the angle between your hips and thighs has been very tight during the ride, so your hip flexors will be a bit shocked about suddenly straightening out for the run.
- Try to run at the same high cadence as you had on the ride, so if you did 90rpm on the bike, aim to run at 90 strides per minute (count how many times your right foot strikes the ground in a minute). This is something you should try in the brick or running sessions in training, but don't panic if you can't manage it – your main priority is to enjoy the race! A high running cadence is an efficient way of increasing speed – your instinct is probably to increase stride length to get more speed, but this uses a lot of energy and can result in overstriding and injury.

Your first few minutes of running off the bike may be a bit slower than your usual pace but, after that, try to maintain this cadence throughout the run, unless you plan to walk-run.

Quick tips

Tuck the zip cord on your wetsuit into the back of your swimming cap. It will make it easier to find after the swim.

Don't put your sunglasses on until last – they often steam up because you're wet and you won't be able to see what you're doing!

If your cycling shoes have movable insoles, glue them down. This lessens the chance of them sliding about when you're putting your feet in.

○ ○ ○ Now you've read about how to perfect every aspect of your training, it's time to tackle the training plans. In association with top Olympic coach Bill Black, we've come up with three plans to suit every level of fitness and ambition. We've also devised a complementary plan of resistance moves and core training to ensure you're 100% race-fit.

11
tri in ten

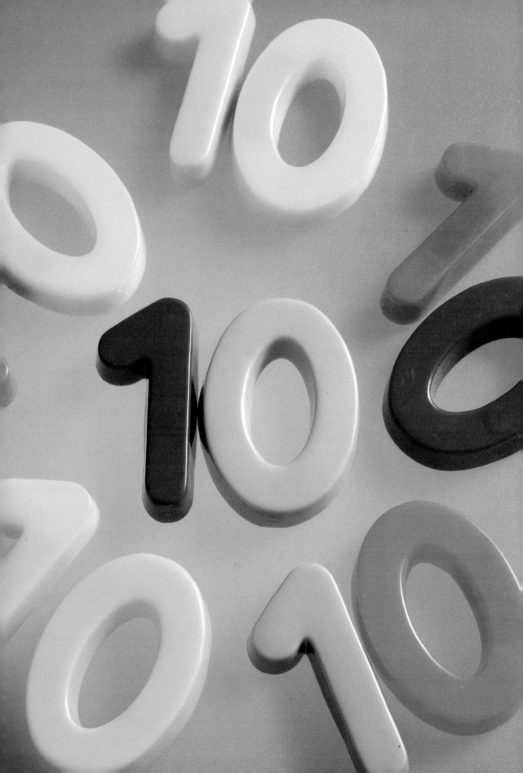

Choosing a plan

If you're not sure where to start, the guides below should help you to establish which of our training plans is best suited to your fitness level. If you're not confident you can match the requirements for the Super-Sprint plan, we've designed a four-week pre-training plan (see below) to help you get ready for the Super-Sprint plan.

To start on the plans, you must be able to:

Super-Sprint plan
- Run for 1 minute, walk for 1 minute for a total of 20 minutes.
- Swim 50m without stopping.
- Cycle at an easy pace for 30 minutes.

Sprint plan
- Run for 30 minutes without stopping.
- Swim 500m without stopping.
- Cycle at an easy pace for 45 minutes.

Olympic plan
- Run for 45 minutes without stopping.
- Swim 800m without stopping.
- Cycle at an easy pace for 60 minutes.

Four-week pre-training plan for real beginners

Follow this plan if you are not yet confident you're fit enough to start the Super-Sprint plan.

Weeks 1 and 2
- Swim: 300m twice a week, with a 10-second rest every 25m
- Bike: 20 minutes at a slow pace twice a week
- Run: 15 minutes jog-walk twice a week (jog for 40 seconds, then walk for 30 seconds, and repeat)

Weeks 3 and 4
- Swim: 300m twice a week, with a 15-second rest every 50m
- Bike: 30 minutes at a slow pace twice a week.
- Run: 20 minutes jog-walk twice a week (jog for 60 seconds, then walk for 60 seconds, and repeat)

The training plans explained

The plans are designed to get you fit for triathlon in the minimum time possible, with varied and easy-to-follow training sessions.

We wrote the plans in collaboration with Olympic triathlon coach Bill Black, a guru in the world of triathlon. All three plans refer to the specific swim, bike and run training sessions we mention in our skills sections. Although they are optional, we strongly recommend that you incorporate the core and body conditioning programmes (see pages 162–5). These should boost your performance in all three disciplines, as well as making you less liable to injury.

Of course, it goes without saying that you should warm up before each training session (see pages 56–7), warm down after, and always stretch. The stretching programme on pages 60–7 was designed specifically with triathletes in mind, so you have no excuse!

The most important thing is that you enjoy the programme. We've tried to keep it varied and pack as much as possible into short sessions, so you don't get bored. Feel free to shake up the order of sessions if you need to. Just be sure to allow yourself adequate rest, and try to avoid doing too much of one discipline on consecutive days.

There are time-trial tests in the Sprint and Olympic plans so you can chart your progress as you speed up. These are not recommended if you're following the Super-Sprint plan, although see page 166 to help you to chart your progress.

Short of time?

The most important sessions in all the plans are the endurance rides and runs. If you have a really busy week and can't fit in every training session, make sure you don't miss out on these. To ensure you complete as many sessions as possible, though, we recommend copying them into your diary, so you can tick them off as you go. We have assumed that race day will be a Sunday (most triathlons are held on Sundays, though not all), but you can adapt your final week's training accordingly if your race day is different. Good luck!

Super-Sprint plan

	Monday	Tuesday	Wednesday	
Week 1	Endurance run (20 min). Jog 1 min, walk 1 min + core moves (15 min optional)	Swim drills (300m total)	Resistance moves (15 min optional) REST	
Week 2	Endurance run (20 min). Jog 90 sec, walk 1 min + core moves (15 min optional)	Swim drills (300m total)	Resistance moves (15 min optional) REST	
Week 3	Endurance run (20 min). Jog 2 min, walk 1 min + core moves (15 min optional)	Swim drills (300m total)	Resistance moves (15 min optional) REST	
Week 4	Endurance run (25 min). Jog 3 min, walk 1 min + core moves (15 min optional)	Swim drills (300m total)	Resistance moves (15 min optional) REST	
Week 5	Endurance run (25 min). Jog 3 min, walk 1 min + core moves (15 min optional)	Swim drills (400m total)	Resistance moves (15 min optional) REST	

Thursday	Friday	Saturday	Sunday
Easy ride (20 min) + core moves (15 min optional)	Recovery swim (30 min). Break every 50m for 15 sec if you need to	Endurance ride (30 min)	Resistance moves (15 min optional) REST
Cadence ride (20 min) + core moves (15 min optional)	Recovery swim (30 min). Break every 50m for 15 sec if you need to	BRICK ride 15 min + 10-min tempo run (jog 90 sec, walk 1 min)	Resistance moves (15 min optional) REST
BRICK ride 25 min + 15-min tempo run (jog 2 min, walk 1 min)	Recovery swim (30 min). Break every 75m for 20 sec if you need to	Endurance ride (30 min)	Resistance moves (15 min optional) REST
Cadence ride (20 min) + core moves (15 min optional)	Recovery swim (30 min). Break every 100m for 25 sec if you need to	BRICK ride 20 min + 10-min tempo run (jog 3 min, walk 1 min)	Resistance moves (15 min optional) REST
BRICK ride 30 min + 15-min tempo run (jog 3.5 min, walk 1 min)	Recovery swim (30 min). Break every 150m for 25 sec if you need to	Endurance ride (35 min)	Resistance moves (15 min optional) REST

Super-Sprint plan

	Monday	Tuesday	Wednesday	
Week 6	Endurance run (30 min). Jog 4 min, walk 1 min + core moves (15 min optional)	Swim drills (400m total)	Resistance moves (15 min optional) REST	
Week 7	Endurance run (30 min). Jog 4 min, walk 1 min + core moves (15 min optional)	Swim drills (400m total)	Resistance moves (15 min optional) REST	
Week 8	Endurance run (35 min). Jog 5 min, walk 1 min	Swim drills (500m total)	Resistance moves (15 min optional) REST	
Week 9	Endurance run (25 min). Jog 5 min, walk 1 min	Swim drills (500m total)	Resistance moves (15 min optional) REST	
Week 10	Endurance run (15 min). Jog 5 min, walk 1 min	Swim drills (500m total)	REST	

Thursday	Friday	Saturday	Sunday
Cadence ride (25 min) + core moves (15 min optional)	Recovery swim (30 min). Break every 200m for 25 sec if you need to	BRICK ride 25 min + 15-min tempo run (jog 4 min, walk 1 min)	Resistance moves (15 min optional) REST
BRICK ride 35 min + 20-min tempo run (jog 4 min, walk 1 min)	Recovery swim (30 min). Break every 400m for 30 sec if you need to	Endurance ride (45 min)	Resistance moves (15 min optional) REST
Cadence ride (25 min) + core moves (15 min optional)	Recovery swim (30 min) with one break halfway through	BRICK ride 30 min + 15-min tempo run (jog 5 min, walk 1 min)	Resistance moves (15 min optional) REST
Cadence ride (30 min) + core moves (15 min optional)	Endurance ride (50 min)	BRICK ride 35 min + 15-min tempo run (jog 5 min, walk 1 min)	Resistance moves (15 min optional) REST
Easy ride (10–15 min)	REST	Easy ride (10 min) 5 min jog	RACE!

Sprint plan

	Monday	Tuesday	Wednesday	
Week 1	Endurance run (30 min) + core moves (15 min optional)	Swim drills (500m total) + 500m slow swim	Resistance moves (15 min optional) REST	
Week 2	Endurance run (30 min) + core moves (15 min optional)	Swim drills (500m total) + endurance ride (40 min)	Resistance moves (15 min optional) REST	
Week 3	Endurance run (35 min) + core moves (15 min optional)	Swim drills (600m total) + 500m slow swim	Resistance moves (15 min optional) REST	
Week 4	Endurance run (35 min) + core moves (15 min optional)	Swim drills (600m total) + endurance ride (40 min)	Resistance moves (15 min optional) REST	
Week 5	Endurance run (40 min) + core moves (15 min optional)	Swim drills (750m total) + 500m slow swim	Resistance moves (15 min optional) REST	

Thursday	Friday	Saturday	Sunday
3K running time trial + core moves (15 min optional)	**⅔ race distance swim time trial** interval swim (15 min)	**10K ride time trial**	Resistance moves (15 min optional) + endurance ride (30–45 min)
Cadence ride (20 min) + core moves (15 min optional)	Interval swim (20 min)	BRICK ride 20 min + 10-min tempo run	Resistance moves (15 min optional) + endurance ride (30–45 min)
Interval run (20 min) + core moves (15 min optional)	Interval swim (20 min)	BRICK ride 20 min + 10-min tempo run	Resistance moves (15 min optional) + endurance ride (30–45 min)
10K ride time trial + core moves (15 min optional)	Interval swim (20 min)	BRICK ride 20 min + 10-min tempo run	Resistance moves (15 min optional) + endurance ride (30–45 min)
3K running time trial + core moves (15 min optional)	**⅔ race distance swim time trial** + interval swim (15 mins)	BRICK ride 25 min + 10-min tempo run	Resistance moves (15 min optional) + endurance ride (30–45 min)

Sprint plan

	Monday	Tuesday	Wednesday	
Week 6	Endurance run (40 min) + core moves (15 min optional)	Swim drills (750m total) + endurance ride (40 min)	Resistance moves (15 min optional) REST	
Week 7	Endurance run (45 min) + core moves (15 min optional)	Swim drills (750m total) + 400m slow swim	Resistance moves (15 min optional) REST	
Week 8	Endurance run (45 min) + core moves (15 min optional)	Swim drills (1000m total) + endurance ride (40 min)	Resistance moves (15 min optional) REST	
Week 9	Endurance run (50 min) + core moves (15 min optional)	Swim drills (750m total)	Resistance moves (15 min optional) REST	
Week 10	Endurance run (30 min) + core moves (15 min optional)	Swim drills (500m total)	REST	

Thursday	Friday	Saturday	Sunday
Cadence ride (25 min) + core moves (15 min optional)	Interval swim (25 min)	BRICK ride 30 min + 15-min tempo run	Resistance moves (15 min optional) + endurance ride (30–45 min)
Interval run (25 min) + core moves (15 min optional)	Interval swim (25 min)	BRICK ride 30 min + 15-min tempo run	Resistance moves (15 min optional) + endurance ride (30–45 min)
10K ride time trial + core moves (15 min optional)	Interval swim (30 min)	BRICK ride 35 min + 20-min tempo run	Resistance moves (15 min optional) + endurance ride (30–45 min)
3K running time trial + core moves (15 min optional)	**⅔ race distance swim time trial** + interval swim (15 min)	BRICK ride 30 min + 15-min tempo run	Resistance moves (15 min optional) + endurance ride (30 min)
Easy ride (10–15 min) + easy run (5–10 min)	REST	Easy ride (10 min) + easy run (5 min)	RACE!

Olympic plan

	Monday	Tuesday	Wednesday	
Week 1	Resistance moves (15 min optional) REST	**5K running time trial** + core moves (15 min optional)	Swim drills (1000m total)	
Week 2	Resistance moves (15 min optional) REST	Interval run (25min)	BRICK ride 30 min + 10-min tempo run	
Week 3	Resistance moves (15 min optional) REST	Hill run. 10 min endurance pace + short hill repeats x 8, another 10 min endurance pace + core moves (15 min optional)	BRICK ride 40 min + 10-min tempo run	
Week 4	Resistance moves (15 min optional) REST	Interval run (30 min) Swim drills (1200m total)	BRICK ride 45 min + 15-min tempo run + resistance moves (15 min optional)	
Week 5	Resistance moves (15 min optional) REST	Swim drills (1200m total) + 500m slow swim	BRICK ride 50 min + 10-min tempo run	

Thursday	Friday	Saturday	Sunday
Hill run. 10 min endurance pace + short hill repeats x 6, another 10 min endurance pace + resistance moves (15 min optional)	**750m swim time trial** + interval swim (15 min)	Endurance run (45 min) + core moves (15 min optional)	**20K ride time trial**
Interval swim (6 x 200m repeats) + resistance moves (15 min optional)	Cadence ride (30 min) + core moves (15 min optional) + swim drills (1000m total)	Endurance run (50 min) + core moves (15 min optional)	Endurance ride (60 min)
Cadence ride (35 min) + interval swim (7 x 200m repeats) + resistance moves (15 min optional)	Swim drills (1200m total) + 500m slow swim	Endurance run (60 min) + core moves (15 min optional)	Endurance ride (70 min)
Interval swim (7 x 200m repeats) + core moves (15 min optional)	**20K ride time trial**	Endurance run (60 min) + core moves (15 min optional)	Endurance ride (75 min)
5K running time trial + core moves (15 min optional)	**750m swim time trial** + cadence ride (35 min) + resistance moves (optional)	Endurance run (60 min) + core moves (15 min optional)	Endurance ride (80 min)

Olympic plan

	Monday	Tuesday	Wednesday	
Week 6	Resistance moves (15 min optional) REST	Cadence ride (25 min) + interval swim (8 x 200m repeats) + core moves (15 min optional)	BRICK ride 60 min + 10 min tempo run	
Week 7	Resistance moves (15 min optional) REST	Cadence ride (35 min) + interval swim (9 sets 200m repeats)	BRICK Ride 60 min + 15-min tempo run + core moves (15 min optional)	
Week 8	Resistance moves (15 min optional) REST	Swim drills (1750m total) + **20K ride time trial** + core moves (15 min optional)	BRICK ride 70 min + 15-min tempo run	
Week 9	Resistance moves (15 min optional) REST	**5K running time trial** + Swim drills (1750m total) + core moves (15 min optional)	BRICK ride 60 min + 20-min tempo run	
Week 10	REST	BRICK ride 20 min + 10-min tempo run	Swim drills (1750m total)	

Thursday	Friday	Saturday	Sunday
Hill run. 10 min endurance pace + short hill repeats x 8 + 10 more mins endurance pace + resistance moves (15 min optional)	Swim drills (1500m total)	Endurance run (50 min) + core moves (15 min optional)	Endurance ride (95 min)
Interval run (30 min)	Swim drills (1500m total) + 400m Recovery swim + resistance moves (15 min optional)	Endurance run (70 min) + core moves (15 min optional)	Endurance ride (1 hour 45 min)
Hill run. 10 min endurance pace + hill repeats x 10, another 10 min endurance pace + resistance moves (15 min optional)	Interval swim (10 x 200m repeats)	Endurance run (80 min) + core moves (15 min optional)	Endurance ride (90 min)
Cadence ride (40 min) + resistance moves (15 min optional)	**750m swim time trial** + interval swim (5 x 200m repeats)	Endurance run (60 min) + core moves (15 min optional)	Endurance ride (80 min)
REST Or 20-min easy ride	REST	Easy ride 15 min + 10 min easy run	RACE!

Playing to your strengths

It's very rare to find someone who's brilliant at all three triathlon sports – you've probably got more strength and skill in at least one of them. This means that while you're training, it can be tempting to do more of the sport you're good at and avoid your weaker ones. Why flounder about in the pool when you could be running effortlessly through the park? Why huff up hills on the bike when you could be doing 30 lengths of crawl without batting an eyelid? The answer is this – by focusing on your strengths, you're not strengthening your weaknesses.

'My advice would be to start focusing immediately on your weaker discipline in the early weeks of training,' says Chris Volley, lead triathlon coach at Team Bath High-Performance Centre. 'That way, you can try to bring them closer to the level of your stronger disciplines, then the rest of your training can be balanced. So, if you're an excellent swimmer but a weak cyclist, maybe swap a few of your swim sessions in the early weeks of training to bike sessions and really focus on improving your technique.'

Mix and match
'Another way to motivate yourself would be to bring elements of your strong discipline into your weak one,' says Volley. If you're a good runner, swap a few of your lengths in the pool with aqua jogging (running up and down in the pool). Or if you don't like resistance work but like cycling, use one of your bike rides as a resistance session for your legs by using high gears and hills (don't do this too often, though, as it can lead to overstressing the knees if you don't allow yourself adequate recovery).

Balance it out
Once you feel more confident on your weaker discipline, make sure you return to a balanced training programme. 'The thing to remember when you're tempted to do more of one discipline is that they all benefit each other,' says Volley. 'For example, swimming can help to improve your aerobic fitness, which makes running easier, and cycling can help you to be a faster runner by strengthening your leg muscles.'

They also each have distinct benefits – cycling maintains fitness without taxing your legs in the way that running does, swimming strengthens your entire body with very little impact, and running improves your cardiovascular fitness like nothing else. You're much less likely to get an injury if you keep a good balance between the three.

If you could focus on one thing...

It goes without saying that nothing replaces variety in training for each discipline, but there are things you can prioritise within the discipline you're not so good at, according to Volley. Here are the golden rules for making each one a little easier come race day.

Swimming

Technique is the key for swimming. Water can be very unforgiving, so your priority should be to learn how to move through it as efficiently as possible. This doesn't mean having 100% perfect technique, but you should feel that you're getting something back for the effort you're putting in. Even if you're superfit, swimming is hard work if your technique is lacking. Doing drills, joining a tri club, or taking lessons are all good ways to improve your technique.'

Cycling

Cadence is the key for triathlon cycling. If you manage to master maintaining a high cadence on the bike, you're going to have a much nicer run. High cadence uses your heart and lung system, whereas low cadence uses your power and muscular strength, leaving little energy in your legs when you get off the bike. See page 106 for more on cadence and good technique.

Running

Obviously, fitness counts for a lot in running, but make sure you're familiar with the sensations of a triathlon run by doing brick sessions. The jelly-leg feeling can really throw you if you're a beginner, but it won't if you've experienced it in training.

On race day

Even after several weeks or months of training, you're still likely to be better at one or two of the disciplines, so should you go hell for leather in one discipline to make up for your weaker ones? The answer, according to Volley, is no. 'Instead, enjoy the discipline you're good at – if you go too fast, you'll crash and burn for the following disciplines and end up with a slower total time,' he says.

'For example, if you're a good swimmer and decide to give everything you've got to make up for a weaker ride, what may actually happen is that you'll do an even slower ride than usual because you have nothing left. The same goes for the run, even though it's last. If you set out at a sprint to make up for a weaker swim and bike, you're likely to end up being slower than if you set off at a strong, steady pace. This is not to say that you shouldn't play to your strengths at all – it's only natural you'll do that to some extent. But keep a lid on it or you won't enjoy the race!'

The core programme

In addition to your swimming, cycling and running training, most coaches agree that all good triathletes need a programme of core conditioning to prevent injury, correct postural imbalance and improve form. John Sullivan of TriCampUK.com, who devised the following exercises, says, 'A strong core is crucial for triathletes; working to strengthen it will benefit every aspect of your training.'

Getting started

Unless otherwise stated, do two sets of eight repetitions for each exercise. Build up to two sets of 15 repetitions as you get stronger. You should aim to complete this set of exercises two or three times a week. It should take you no more than 15 minutes each time.

You will need

- An exercise or yoga mat
- A set of hand weights (1.3–2.25kg (3–5lb) or heavy enough to leave you feeling fatigued after each set)
- A resistance band
- A Swiss ball

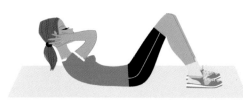

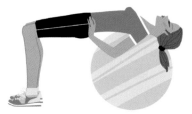

Torso raise

1. Lie on your back with your knees bent. Place your hands behind your head.
2. Slowly raise your shoulders off the floor, contracting your abdominal muscles for a count of two. Roll back down slowly as you release.

Back bridge

1. Sit on a Swiss ball. Walk your legs forwards as you roll the ball up your back towards your shoulders. Stop when you are in a bridge position, with your knees bent at 90°.
2. Press your hips up as you rest your shoulders on the ball. Hold for 30 seconds, then roll back again to sitting. Aim to hold for up to 60 seconds as you get stronger.

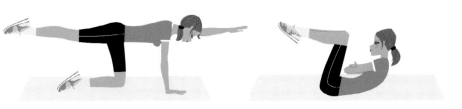

Superman

1. Place your hands and knees on the mat, with your back straight.
2. Stretch your right arm out in front, then your left leg straight behind. Engage your abdominals to hold the position with control. Hold for a count of two.
3. Return to all fours, then repeat with your left arm and right leg.

Leg crunch

1. Lie on your back with your knees bent, arms crossed.
2. Engage your abdominals and lift your knees slowly, crunching them in towards your chest. Return your legs to the mat slowly and with control. To make this exercise more challenging, straighten your legs as you lower them.

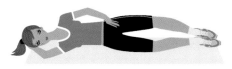

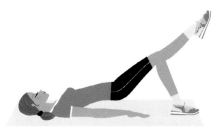

Clam raise

1. Lie on your right side, with your knees bent and heels together, in line with your spine.
2. Engage your left glute (bottom muscle), and raise your left knee towards the ceiling, keeping your heels together. Complete one set of eight repetitions, then turn over to the other side and repeat.

Half-bridge extension

1. Lie on your back with your knees bent and your feet hip-width apart. Engage your abdominal muscles and raise your body, resting your weight on your shoulders.
2. Tuck in your pelvis and keep your abdominal muscles engaged as you slowly extend your right leg straight out. Return your leg to the mat with control before repeating with the left leg. This is one repetition.

The body conditioning programme

Regular resistance training can help to ensure that all your muscles are in optimum condition to support your training regime. It has been found to increase lean muscle mass significantly – great news for triathletes. John Sullivan says that just a few simple moves performed twice a week will make a real difference. As with the core exercises, unless otherwise specified do two sets of eight repetitions for each exercise, building up to two sets of 15 repetitions as you get stronger.

Squat

1. Stand with your feet hip-width apart. With arms folded, bend your knees and lower your bottom towards the floor until you reach a 'sitting' position. Check that your knees stay in line with your ankles.
2. Push through your legs and bottom to return to a standing position.

Weighted lunge

1. Stand with your feet hip-width apart, holding a weight in each hand.
2. Step your right foot forwards about an arm-length away. Lower your body into a lunge, but don't let your left knee touch the mat.
3. Push up, returning to your start position, and repeat on the other side.

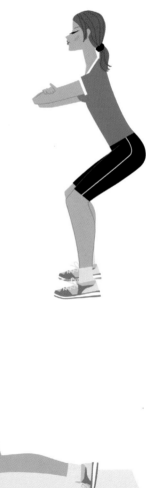

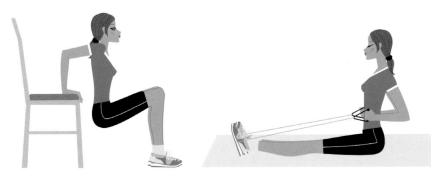

Triceps dip

1. Sit on a bench or chair with your hands on either side of your hips, fingers facing forwards.
2. Lift your hips forward off the bench or chair, and bend your elbows to lower your bottom. Bend your arms to 90°.
3. Push back up without locking your elbows.

Box press-up

1. Place your hands and knees on the mat, with your back straight, your hands underneath your shoulders, and fingers facing forwards.
2. Bend your elbows and lower your chest towards the floor, making a right angle with your arms, until no lower than 5cm (2in) from the mat.
3. Push back up, feeling the work in your chest, arms and shoulders. To make this more challenging, straighten your legs, resting on your toes as you press-up.

Seated row

1. Sit on the floor, with your knees bent and your back straight. Hold a resistance band around your feet; your hands should be in line with your knees and your arms shoulder-width apart.
2. Relax your shoulders and look straight ahead. Breathe in and then breathe out, pulling the resistance band towards you. As you pull, bend your elbows, straighten your legs, and squeeze your shoulder blades together. Keep your abdominal muscles engaged throughout. Return to the starting position.

Note: The wider apart your arms, the more this exercise works your chest. The closer together, the more it works your triceps.

My triathlon journal

Over the next 10 pages, we've created a fill-in 10-week journal, designed to be used in conjunction with the three training plans in the Tri in Ten chapter. Record every session you complete, along with how it felt. If you have time, note down what you eat every day and make a note of your energy levels and mood. Don't forget to reward yourself, too!

Week 1	What I did:	What I ate:	How I felt:
Monday			
Tuesday			
Wednesday			
Thursday			
Friday			
Saturday			
Sunday			

❝ What you dream you can do, begin it! Boldness has genius, power and magic in it. ❞
Goethe, writer and philosopher

Week 2	What I did:	What I ate:	How I felt:
Monday			
Tuesday			
Wednesday			
Thursday			
Friday			
Saturday			
Sunday			

66 The fearless are merely fearless. People who act in spite of their fear are truly brave. 99

James A. Lafond-Lewis, writer

Week 3	What I did:	What I ate:	How I felt:
Monday			
Tuesday			
Wednesday			
Thursday			
Friday			
Saturday			
Sunday			

66 Make the most of yourself,
for that is all there is of you. 99
Ralph Waldo Emerson, philosopher and writer

Week 4	What I did:	What I ate:	How I felt:
Monday			
Tuesday			
Wednesday			
Thursday			
Friday			
Saturday			
Sunday			

66Life shrinks and expands in proportion to one's courage.99

Anaïs Nin, writer

Week 5	What I did:	What I ate:	How I felt:
Monday			
Tuesday			
Wednesday			
Thursday			
Friday			
Saturday			
Sunday			

66 Today I do the things other people won't, so tomorrow I can do the things other people can't. **99**

Anon

Week 6	What I did:	What I ate:	How I felt:
Monday			
Tuesday			
Wednesday			
Thursday			
Friday			
Saturday			
Sunday			

66 Pain is temporary. It may last a minute, or an hour, or a day, or a year, but eventually it will subside and something else will take its place. If I quit, however, it lasts for ever. **99**

Lance Armstrong, cyclist

Week 7	What I did:	What I ate:	How I felt:
Monday			
Tuesday			
Wednesday			
Thursday			
Friday			
Saturday			
Sunday			

❝It's not the size of the dog in the fight but the size of the fight in the dog that counts.❞

Mark Twain, writer

Week 8	What I did:	What I ate:	How I felt:
Monday			
Tuesday			
Wednesday			
Thursday			
Friday			
Saturday			
Sunday			

❝Be the change you wish to see.❞
Mahatma Ghandi, statesman

Week 9	What I did:	What I ate:	How I felt:
Monday			
Tuesday			
Wednesday			
Thursday			
Friday			
Saturday			
Sunday			

❝Eighty per cent of success is showing up.❞
Woody Allen, writer and filmmaker

Week 10	What I did:	What I ate:	How I felt:
Monday			
Tuesday			
Wednesday			
Thursday			
Friday			
Saturday			
Sunday			

66 We never know how high we are

'till we are called to rise. **99**

Emily Dickinson, poet

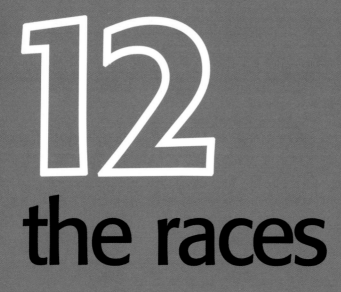

Ready to get your cheque book out and sign up to that race? Before you do, we've devised a quiz to help you to identify the perfect event for you. There's a list of tris to try, and pointers on how to beat the racing pitfalls (as well as tips from the pros for race day). Last, but not least, we've created a race-day checklist to cover all the kit you might need.

12
the races

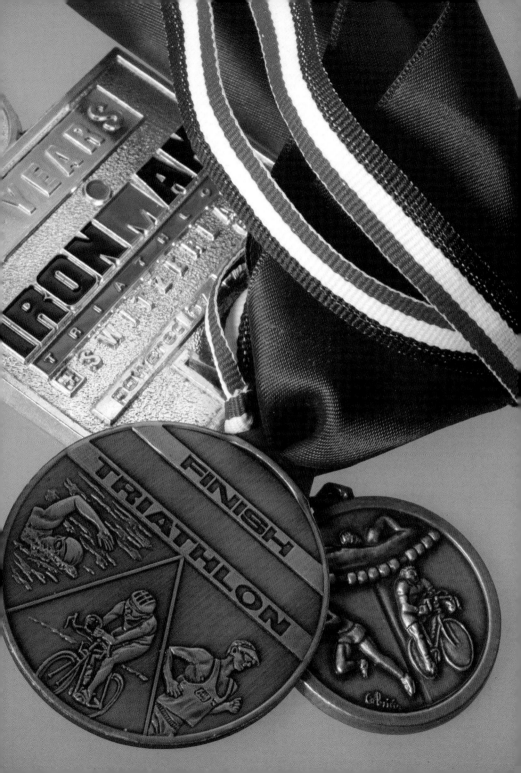

Quiz: What's your race personality?

Before you sign up for a tri, it's important to establish exactly what you want from your racing experience. There's such a huge variety of triathlon events on offer, there's something for everyone. Relay team races, where you compete as a team with a different person doing each different element of the course, is a good way to start triathlon. There are also adventure triathlons, where you'll be mountain biking and running over rugged cross-country trails. There are pool-swims and sea-swims, seriously sporty races and 'fun' ones, so there's sure to be a race that inspires you. Do our quiz to work out which you should choose.

Your idea of a great run is:

A: A straight, flat road stretching into the distance – the perfect time to enjoy your own thoughts, and the sound of your feet hitting the tarmac.
B: A muddy, off-road challenge where you don't know what's coming round the next bend.
C: Fast and furious. You love to run with a purpose, and get a buzz out of passing other runners on your way.
D: A trot around your local park with a friend on a sunny day.

Your partner has booked a surprise activity for your birthday. You're overjoyed when you find out it is:

A: A long, rambling cliff-top walk, so you can work up an appetite before your pub lunch.
B: A canyoning trip. The combination of scrambling up muddy banks, plunging into fast-flowing rivers and discovering gorgeous scenery is your idea of heaven.
C: Go-karting; your competitive instinct will kick in and you plan to win.
D: A hot-air balloon ride followed by a picnic – romantic and a chance to spend some time together.

At school the sport you excelled at was:

A: Swimming. You enjoyed perfecting your technique.
B: Anything adventurous and outdoorsy: orienteering, climbing, cross-country running.
C: Sports that pitted you against an opponent: tennis, athletics, Judo…
D: Netball or football – all your best friends were in the team, so you enjoyed the social element.

The point of life is:

A: The journey. You believe in making the most of every moment, rather than focusing on the end-point.
B: To adjust to eternal change: A life well lived is a constant (but enjoyable) challenge.
C: To be the best you can be. Natural selection means that the winner takes all.
D: To build strong relationships with your friends, family and neighbours so you can support one another.

Your motto is:

A: 'Keep on running'
B: 'Bring it on!'
C: 'Don't stop till you get enough'
D: 'There's no I in "team"'

Imagine your perfet gym. It would be:

A: Not too crowded, with no time restrictions on the cardio machines; you hate feeling rushed and can't bear having to queue.

B: Impossible. You hate gyms – you'd rather be outdoors.

C: Packed with super-fit, toned and beautiful people to inspire you to raise your game.

D: Friendly. Full of like-minded people without any attitude.

Mostly As: You live for the moment

When it comes to sport, you're not concerned about your time, or pushing yourself to the limit. Your objective is to enjoy what you're doing. Exercise is your 'me' time. Choose a race somewhere beautiful so you can savour every moment of the course. You naturally tend towards longer-distance events, so if you're already very fit, an Olympic-distance triathlon would be ideal.

Mostly Bs: You're a fan of the great outdoors

You're perfectly suited to rough and rugged challenges, so opt for an off-road race with a cross-country course, and an open-water swim. Pool swims and road racing could leave you cold.

Mostly Cs: You're the competitive type

You have a low boredom-threshold, and crave competition in every aspect of your life. You can't set out for a casual run with a friend without secretly hoping you'll prove yourself to be fitter and faster than them. Pick a race that's fast, such as a Sprint or Super-Sprint.

Mostly Ds: You're a sociable people-person

As far as you're concerned, sport is a social event. You enjoy activities far more when you're part of a team. Enter a short triathlon with a group of friends and agree to stick together, or enter a race as a relay team, with one of you doing the swim, another the cycle and another the run.

179

Races to tri

There's nothing quite as inspiring as signing up for a race and paying your entry fee. It gives you a goal to aim for, and will act as the ultimate training incentive. Here are a few of the best, from those to sign up for immediately to the world's most famous (and notorious!)...

Sign up now

These races offer shorter distances and are very welcoming to first-time entrants – we can vouch for it!

The Michelob Ultra London Triathlon

The biggest triathlon in the world, with more than 11,000 competitors, this is a great race. Choose from Super-Sprint, Sprint or Olympic distance. The course runs around London's Docklands area.
www.thelondontriathlon.com
Super-Sprint (400m swim, 10K bike, 2.5K run)
Sprint (750m swim, 20K bike, 5K run)
Olympic (1500m swim, 40K bike, 10K run)

Timex Women's Only Triathlon

Friendly and non-intimidating, this race takes place in and around Dorney Lake in Eton. Choose from three distances:
Novice (200m swim, 5K bike, 2.5K run)
Sprint (400m swim, 20K bike, 5K run)
Challenge (800m swim, 30K bike, 7.5K run) www.humanrace.co.uk

The Stratford 220 Triathlon

The UK's biggest pool-based swim, this is an ideal race for beginners. Set in the pretty town of Stratford-upon-Avon, there are three distances to choose from:
Fun (200m swim, 23K bike, 2.5K run)
Sprint (400m swim, 23K bike, 5K run)
Relay (where you work in a team with a different competitor for each leg) (400m swim, 23K bike, 5K run).
www.fun2tri.co.uk

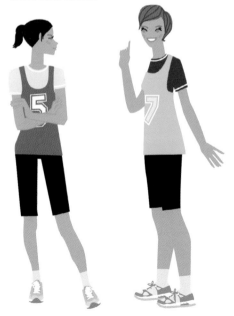

Sign up in the future

These are the races to aim for when you want something more demanding.

UK Ironman 70.3

This half-Ironman race, usually set in a stunning rural location, is ideal for triathletes who have done an Olympic-distance event and are craving something more challenging distance-wise. It requires a 1.2mile swim, 56 mile bike, and 13.1 mile run. www.ironmanuk.com

XTERRA UK

XTERRA is an international triathlon adventure race series, which combines mountain biking and trail running with open-water swimming for triathletes who like their events muddy. It involves a 1500m swim, 34K bike, and 10K run.

The UK race is based in the Vale of Neath, South Wales, but XTERRA runs races everywhere from Argentina to Japan, so if you fancy signing up for one of its international events there are plenty to choose from. www.xterraplanet.com

In your dreams

For those in search of a challenge, here are some 'once-in-a-lifetime' races to inspire you.

Escape from Alcatraz

This race, which sets off from the infamous island off the San Francisco coast, has a reputation as one of the toughest in the world. It requires a 1.5 mile

swim, 18 mile bike, and 8 mile run. It's notoriously challenging, thanks to the freezing swim, technically tricky cycle course, and sandy run. www.escapefromalcatraztriathlon.com

Ironman Hawaii

Probably the most famous triathlon in the world and the venue for the Ironman World Championships. The race was started in 1978 by a group of US Navy Seals, and has continued ever since. What makes it unique is that elite athletes compete alongside 200 lucky hopefuls who apply in a ballot. It requires a gruelling 2.4 mile swim, 112 mile bike, and 26.2 mile run. Phew! www.ironman.com

Beat the pitfalls

After months of training, it's easy to get carried away on race day, particularly when there's a lot of adrenaline pumping round your system. Here is our guide to making sure you avoid the common pitfalls that many beginners experience:

THE DANGER: Overdoing it at the start of the race

Many first time triathletes set off too quickly at the start of the swim. 'Particularly because the swim is short, competitive types can blast off at full pelt and forget all about form and pacing,' says swim coach Penny Porter. Before you know it, she says, your technique has gone out of the window. The net result is that your stroke becomes inefficient and you overuse your legs, tiring them before the bike ride. Instead, take a few deep breaths before the start and mentally run through your swimming race plan. Remind yourself of the form pointers you focused on in training, and aim to keep your pace steady and controlled.

THE DANGER: Getting caught in the scrum

Positioning yourself in the right place before you start to swim is crucial. In triathlons strong swimmers 'tend to sprint the first 100 or so metres to get ahead of the pack', says swim coach Helen Gorman. 'If you get caught up in a group of them, they're likely to swim over and under you if you're in the way, which can be frightening.' While researching this book, we lost count of the number of first-time tri-ers who had had this experience. 'My first open-water triathlon swim was

absolutely terrifying,' says Kate Rew, 38. 'I almost had a panic attack in the water – there were men and women swimming under and over me.'

This is easily avoided by starting wide (on the side of the pack) and towards the back. You want to feel comfortable when you leave the water, ready to begin the bike ride with plenty of confidence, so a few extra seconds in the water is a worthwhile price to pay. And if the worst does happen? 'Don't stop,' says triathlon swim coach Liz Scott, 'and focus on the fact that it won't last long – it may take 10 to 15 seconds for the stronger swimmers to pass you, but in the meantime simply focus on your stroke, slow it down, and get control of your own movement until the barrage has passed. It sometimes helps simply to count in your head.'

THE DANGER: Swimming off-course

This is particularly easy to do if you are swimming crawl in open water. The main way to prevent this is to practice sight-swimming as part of your training. Whatever you do, don't simply keep sight of the swimmer in front of you and hope for the best, 'because there's every chance they're headed in the wrong direction, too!' says Gorman. Practise sighting in your training (see page 96) so you're used to it on race day. It might feel awkward at first, but it's essential you stay on course.

THE DANGER: Your bike breaking down

The bike leg is the only one in which you rely on something other than yourself to get you through it. If you've spent months training on your bike, it might be a bit worse for wear, especially if you've neglected to maintain it. The last thing you want after all that training is your bike letting you down, so a pre-race service is a good idea. If you know how to change a punctured inner tube, carry a spare one, tyre levers and a pump with you during the race.

'If you dismantle any part of your bike to get it to the race, make sure you've practised how to put it back together again at the other end,' says elite triathlete Olly Freeman. 'Assemble it carefully when you arrive at the race, even if it's just putting the front wheel back on.' Ride it around to check that everything is in working order and check the tyres for anything sticking into them, such as stones.

Also, while you want your tyres to be pumped up for optimum performance, 'don't pump them fully until just before you start if it's a hot day', says Freeman. 'If you leave your bike in transition for ages with fully pumped tyres, the heat will cause the air to expand and could blow your tyre.'

THE DANGER: Forgetting your technique

In all the excitement of race day, it's easy to set out on the bike and forget everything you've learnt about a steady pace and good technique. 'Remember to have your bike ready in an easy gear out of transition. If you can, try to see what the opening half-mile looks like beforehand so you know what to expect,' advises Chris Chamberlin, an exercise physiologist at Royal Holloway, University of London, who specialises in triathlon. 'If you go straight up a hill or round sharp corners in the wrong gear, you'll fatigue yourself very quickly.'

Don't worry about what speed other competitors are doing – focus on your own race, settle into a pace you know you can sustain, and 'remember to keep up as high a cadence as possible by using your gears,' says Chamberlin. Unless you're an elite athlete, people will overtake you, but don't lose heart. It's your race and your achievement, so just enjoy!

THE DANGER: Getting a time penalty

'The bike leg is a prime place for picking up time penalties (or even disqualification!),' says Peter Holmes, of the British Triathlon Federation, 'so read your rules carefully.' The absolute essentials are having your helmet done up before you touch the bike in T1 and keeping it fastened until you put your bike back; not drafting other competitors (unless it's a draft-legal race); observing the mount and dismount lines outside the transition area; and replacing your bike properly in its allotted space. Remember that the Highway Code still applies, even in closed-road races – and listen to any instructions or orders issued by marshals on the course.

THE DANGER: Jelly-leg panic

We've said it before, and we'll say it again – that horrible jelly-leg feeling you get in the first part of the run will wear off. It's easy to panic that your muscles haven't got any more to give, but, says Martin Yelling, GB duathlon champion and coach: 'It's simply your legs adjusting to weight-bearing running after the circular, non-weight-bearing motion of cycling.'

THE DANGER: Overstriding

As much of a danger in training as it is on race day, overstriding is a common problem and can lead to injury. It's tempting to think that lengthening your stride is a great way to increase your speed, but it increases the impact on your muscles and joints every time your foot hits the ground. It also means that as your heel strikes the ground in front of your knee (with some force), it actually has a braking effect on your stride. It's the enemy of forefoot running, which is what you should be aiming for. By definition, if you're overstriding you're running on your heels.

Overstriding is a particular danger after the transition from cycling to running, as the sense of slowness you'll feel as a result of the change in pace, coupled with the muscular fatigue from the cycling, can make you feel as if you're taking baby steps. 'The best advice here is simply to trust your training and go carefully,' says Chris Donald, coach for Purple Patch Running.

THE DANGER: Running crossover

Crossover happens when your feet or arms cross over the midline of your body each time you take a step. We mentioned this briefly in the Perfect Form pointers (see page 122), but crossover can slow you down significantly on race day.

How can you tell if you're doing it? Watch where your feet fall and check the way your arms move as you run. To avoid it, 'focus on moving forwards, relax, and swing your arms backwards and forwards, not side to side,' says running coach Malcolm Balk. 'Remember to keep your elbows at a 90° angle to your body, and keep your hips pointing forwards.'

THE DANGER: Lack of transition planning

Transition is straightforward as long as you think about it before the big day. See page 136 for our guidelines on how to ensure it goes without a hitch.

Tips from the professionals

" I've got a special pre-race playlist on my MP3 player, packed with the sort of songs that send shivers down my spine just to hear them! Of course, it's not always necessary – sometimes soaking up the pre-race atmosphere is enough. But it's good to know I have it if I need it.'
Henny Freeman, GB triathlete

'Watch out for negative people. Don't listen to other competitors going on about how much training they've done. Just relax, and focus on giving 100% in your own race.'
Ralph Hydes, triathlon coach and GB competitor

'Get a good night's sleep two nights before the race – so if you're racing on Sunday, make sure you're tucked up early on Friday night. It might sound strange, but physiologically speaking, the benefits of a good night's sleep take 36 hours to take effect, so you'll reap the benefits on race day.'
Chris Donald, running coach and triathlete

'If possible, I like to have cycled the course to ensure I won't be surprised on race day. I also try not to take it too seriously – by race day the serious stuff should already have been planned, trained for, eaten, drunk, massaged, talked over – whatever you need to feel prepared. My motto is: train hard, race easy!'
Fiona Ford, GB triathlon and aquathlon champion

'Plan ahead by writing down a list of everything that could go wrong on race day, from physical tiredness to your goggles being knocked off. Think about how you're going to deal with each one of these distractions if they happen. Knowing you'll be able to fix it whatever happens will put your mind at rest.'
Richard Allen, pro triathlete and coach

'Remind yourself that you've put in the tough work already. On race day, all you need to do is turn up and give it your best. I suffer a lot with nerves, but the one thing that gives me confidence on the day is that I know I've trained my hardest!'
Annie Emmerson, pro duathlete and triathlete

'Don't forget to have fun! Triathlon is a sport – and one that you may have spent hours training for – but ultimately you should be competing for fun. So when you're swimming in a glorious lake, pedalling through stunning countryside or doing those final miles of running, take a moment to reflect on how lucky you are to be part of such a great sport, with so many amazing volunteers who have turned out to support you! Take a moment to smile, wave and enjoy! And give it your all. Pain is temporary, but glory lasts for ever!'
Vanessa Hogg, GB triathlete "

○ ○ ○ For the eight amazing women on the following pages, triathlon is more than just a sport. From battling a disability to overcoming water-phobia, they've beaten the odds and changed their lives for good.

13

we tri'd it

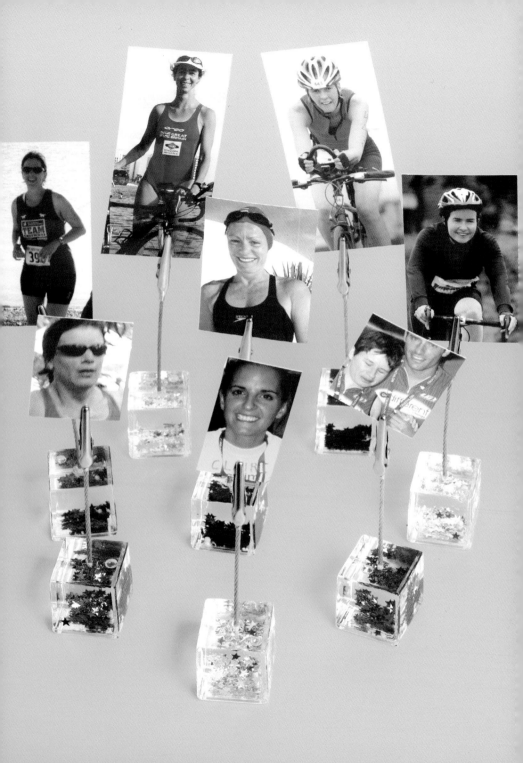

'NOW I CAN COPE WITH ANYTHING LIFE THROWS AT ME'

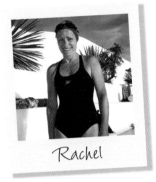

Rachel

For Rachel Black, 54, from London, triathlon changed the way she felt about turning 50 and helped her cope with the strains of caring for her terminally ill mum…

❝ Triathlon has given me an inner and outer strength I never knew I had. I came across the sport quite by accident when I saw an advert for triathlon workshops for beginners on the website of my local running club. I didn't really know what triathlon was but I was looking for new challenges, so I sent an email to the triathlon coach to learn more.

'He responded asking for my swimming, cycling and running experience with best times, requesting I bring my swimsuit, goggles, road bike and "HRM" to the first workshop. I emailed back explaining that the most swimming I'd done in the last 30 years was the occasional dip in hotel pools, I hadn't been near a bike since the age of 14, and that I was very much a fun runner. I also said I didn't own a bike or have a clue what a HRM was, and ended by adding, "… and by the way, I'm 50". I was sure I'd be politely rejected. Instead, he said I was just the sort of person the workshop was aimed at.

'So at 8.30am on a cold October day, 16 of us congregated at a school. We were led to the pool and introduced to Chris, an ex-Olympic swim coach, who told us to swim eight lengths of front crawl. I somehow managed to survive it, although sounded like a 60-a-day smoker. While waiting for the train after the session, I phoned my husband, reporting I'd never felt so exhausted and so exhilarated in my life. That day,

'I'd never felt so exhausted and so exhilarated in my life. That day, my passion for triathlon was born!'

my passion for triathlon was born!

'Over the next five months, I sometimes felt overwhelmed, but John, the coach, was very motivating. I set my sights on the Thames Turbo sprint series and can still recall my pride after finishing my first race. The celebratory bacon sarnie, mug of tea and congratulations from John made me feel like I'd won the lottery.

'After competing in a few sprints, I decided to have a go at Olympic-distance the following year and then a half-Ironman, which I have now achieved. I discovered that the longer distances suit my build and dogged personality best.

'I find triathlon a demanding sport that often requires me to keep going

'It's totally changed my perception of being in my 50s – it's made me embrace, even celebrate, it'

when my body and mind have had enough. Pushing myself to the limits has made me far more confident and courageous. For example, it's totally changed my perception of being in my 50s – it's made me embrace, even celebrate, it. You can't hide your age in a race – I compete with a huge "J" drawn on my leg and arm, which indicates my age group. A lot of the competitors are younger than me and yet they don't pity or ignore me – they express admiration and respect.

'It's also changed my body – I've had far fewer injuries than when I was just running and I now have a strong, muscular, trim physique.

'But, in particular, it's helped me cope with some of the tough times life has thrown my way. It helped me deal with the grief of unwanted childlessness, when my husband decided he didn't want kids. Triathlon also helped me work through the grief I felt after writing my story and interviewing over 60 childless women

for a book I co-wrote on learning to live with childlessness by chance not choice. The long swims, rides and runs give me space to think through all the thoughts and feelings that crowd my mind. But most of all, knowing that I can climb a steep hill without getting off my bike and cope with swimming in rough open water, gives me the confidence that I can cope with whatever else life throws at me.

In 2007, triathlon also enabled me to deal with being key carer to my mother during a long year of suffering from terminal cancer. While she was alive, the training, particularly long early-morning runs along the beach, enabled me to rebalance my mind and process my grief, so that I could return home feeling renewed and able to face another sad and often harrowing day caring for Mum.

Triathlon has filtered through every area of my life – mind, body and spirit. At a time when many of my peers are feeling less confident, less attractive and very middle-aged, I've found a new zest for life. **99**

Rachel's top training tip

'Have your favourite food to hand after a long training session. Thinking of the treat in store can really help you keep going when the going gets tough. My favourites include a toasted bacon buttie or cinnamon bagel with a huge mug of steaming tea.'

'I WAS BARELY WELL ENOUGH TO WATCH A TRIATHLON'

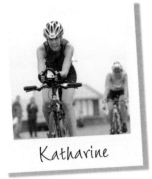

Katharine

Katharine Vile, 36, from southwest London, has had ME (also known as chronic fatigue syndrome) for 17 years. She beat the odds and competed her first triathlon and raised money for the ME Association.

❝ I had always been really sporty throughout my childhood and teens, taking part in tetrathlons (running, horse riding, swimming and shooting), but all that changed in my first year of university when I got glandular fever. I was ill for several months, and then got much worse. I had a blood test, which showed that, despite still feeling ill, I no longer had glandular fever and was diagnosed with ME (myalgic encephalopathy). I had an almost constant temperature and swollen glands, and my muscles were so exhausted and aching that I could hardly walk – all common symptoms of ME, which is often linked to being post-viral.

'I ended up having a break from university as I was too ill to continue. I moved back home to my mother's house and was in bed for long periods. I was mostly too ill to do anything apart from watch a bit of TV or listen to the radio. At times, I felt down because it was hard to be so cut off from life. The break lasted five years in all, until I finally felt well enough to go back and complete my degree.

'When I went back, my illness was manageable, with occasional flare-ups. I still couldn't exercise, but I decided to become a cox for my Oxford college rowing team. It was a way to still be involved in sport without actually doing any exercise!

'I had an almost constant temperature, and my muscles were aching so much I could hardly walk'

'I carried on coxing after university, so I had a lot of friends who were into sport. In 2005, I went to watch one of them do the Michelob Ultra London Triathlon. I was blown away by the atmosphere and remember saying that I wished I could do it too one day. However, I was right in the middle of a really bad relapse and barely felt well enough to watch, let alone take part!

'Over the next few months, I started to come through the relapse and to feel less unwell. The triathlon seed had been planted in my head and I started to think that maybe I could do a triathlon after all. I decided to sign up for the same race my friend had done and see what happened.

'The training was tough at first. I hadn't exercised properly for years and it was a real juggling act. I had to rest for at least a day after a training

'Both my family and I had tears in our eyes as I approached the finish line'

'I had to rest for at least a day after a training session and my glands would always flare up'

session and my glands would always flare up. I built it up slowly and started cycling to work once a week, then twice a week. I was also working full-time, so everything else went out of the window – I didn't have the energy for working, training and socialising, so I virtually ditched the latter to focus on getting fit.

'Thankfully, I had no major relapses during training but then the week before the race, I started to feel bad again. I was so disappointed and almost resigned myself to not being able to do the race. In an attempt to get well enough, I spent the day before the race in bed and it worked. I didn't feel fabulous on the day of the race, but I was well enough to try and I think the adrenaline probably helped!

'I ended up loving the race. The electric atmosphere and the supporters all the way around the course spurred me on and I found it all really exciting. Before I started, I wasn't convinced I'd be able to finish, but I did and coming over the finish line was very emotional. My mother and brother were both there – they had been worried about me doing it, so when they saw me coming towards the finish there were tears in their eyes, as there were in mine! I also raised loads of money for The ME Association, so it was a great day.

'I've definitely got the bug now! I did another triathlon that season and am now part of the Herbalife Triathlon Academy, which is giving me guidance on training and nutrition. I still have bad times with the ME, but am hoping to get a better balance in my training this year, so that I don't have so many setbacks in my health. I think that I will always have the ME, but when I'm lucky enough to be in good health, I can't think of anything better to be doing than triathlons! 99

Katharine's top training tip
'Always listen to your body – sometimes you need to be tough and push yourself when you'd rather curl up under the duvet, and sometimes you need to let your body dictate. Rest and recovery are just as important as the training.'

'I COULD ONLY DO DOGGY PADDLE, NOW I'M A TRIATHLETE!'

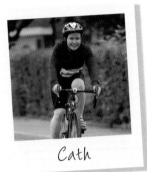

Cath

Cath O'Connor, 34, from Rotherham, was petrified of water, but resolved to conquer her fear. Now she swims with confidence and has competed in an open-water triathlon.

❝ I'd hated the water since I was young. My memories of swimming lessons consist of breathlessly doing doggy paddle while being poked with a stick by the instructor to make me go faster! I left swimming lessons with my 25m doggy-paddle certificate and never went back!

'Amazingly, I managed to avoid exercise until I was 25, when I realised that I should start exercising for the sake of my health (I have exercise-induced asthma and the lung function of a 66-year-old). I bought my first mountain bike for £10 and took up running, both of which I loved. However, I really started to feel held back by not being able to swim. On holiday in Ecuador, everyone waded in and swam in the big rivers that feed the Amazon while I had to paddle around at the edge; in Australia, my friends all went surfing while I watched from the beach.

'Incidents like these built up until one day I decided that I was going to learn to swim before my 30th birthday.

Years of not being able to swim had made me terrified of the water, especially being out of my depth, but I had made my mind up. I found adult swimming lessons at Leeds International Pool and signed up.

'It was a relief when I turned up and found the lessons were in the

'I left swimming lessons with my 25m doggy-paddle certificate and never went back!'

baby pool! The instructor was really kind and encouraging and taught us to feel comfortable putting our faces in the water and breathing out before beginning to teach us breaststroke. Two months later, I had built enough confidence and skill to go in the big 50m pool, although I always swam along the side in case I needed to cough or get my breath back.

'Around this time, a friend started going out with a guy who did triathlons. They went on holiday to

France and she ended up doing a triathlon there – I was so full of admiration as she could barely ride a bike! I thought that if she did it without being great on a bike, then I could do it without being a champion swimmer, so I signed up for a local sprint triathlon with a pool swim.

'Race day came around and I was really nervous as I got into the water, but I focused on staying calm when I

'I let everyone go ahead of me at the start, took my time and loved every minute of it'

got splashed or when people overtook me, and ended up really enjoying it! I did breaststroke the whole way as had no idea how to do crawl. I felt such a huge sense of achievement and loved the whole race.

'After that, I decided that open-water swimming was going to be my next challenge. I joined Sheffield Triathlon Club (STC) and signed up for an open-water session. I've never been so scared as I was before that session – I was so convinced I was going to drown, I took two friends to stand at the side and spot me! I put my wetsuit on and got into the water. It was absolutely freezing and I almost had a panic attack, but a lovely guy called Phil (who introduced himself as Fat Lad) had buddied up with me and, with his encouragement, we happily breaststroked around the lake, way behind everyone else.

'That session inspired me to learn front crawl, so I tried to teach myself with the help of a book and advice

from friends. I found it totally exhausting, so went along to STC swim-training sessions. The coach asked to see my crawl and I knew I was a mass of thrashing limbs, even though I was trying my hardest!

'I spent the next few months learning crawl with the help of a coach and also joined STC's TriNovice team for open-water swimming sessions in a nearby lake. It was too deep to put my feet down, so it was there that I learned how to tread water. This was an absolute revelation to me and finally put to rest any sense of fear or panic about water.

'I set my sights on an open-water triathlon and finally did one in 2006 – a sprint triathlon with a 750m lake swim. I was worried about being kicked, so let everyone go ahead of me at the start, took my time and loved every minute of it. Olympic-distance is next!

'If someone had told me in my early 20s that I'd be doing triathlons, I'd have laughed my head off. Triathlon had always sounded like a superhuman feat to me, but it isn't – it's fun and exciting, and anyone can do it if they give it a try. **99**

Cath's top training tip

'Don't worry about not having the top of the range gear for training or the race. I did my first tri on a borrowed bike, wearing a bikini followed by sweat shirt, cycling shorts and mountain bike shoes, and no-one batted an eyelid!'

'I WANTED TO WEAR THE GREAT BRITAIN KIT'

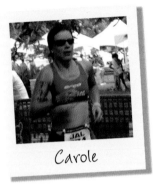

Carole

Full-time mum of three, Carole Heritage, 34, from south London, took on the challenge of a lifetime. She decided that she wanted to represent her country at the ITU Triathlon World Championships.

❝ I had always enjoyed sports at school so when I moved to London in 1997 I joined my local triathlon club to get to know people.

'For the first few years, I'd attend swim sessions and take part in the occasional sprint triathlon. I barely did any training, so they were always a struggle. The club socialising was definitely my strongest discipline!

'I met my husband in 1998, and we had our first son, Lewis, in 2001, followed by Ivor in 2004. I carried on doing sprint triathlons, but with even less training as I was now looking after a baby and toddler full-time.

'When Ivor was six months old, I started to feel that I needed to do something else apart from look after the kids for the sake of my own sanity. Over the years, a few people at my triathlon club had qualified to represent GB in their age group at the ITU Triathlon World Championships (Olympic-distance).

After years of dabbling in triathlon, I decided that I wanted to wear the GB kit and compete for my country!

'This was in October 2004. My husband was very supportive, so I got myself a coach and launched into a training programme. Over the next eight months, I looked after the children all day and then went out training at night. I did this six nights a week plus several hours of cycling at the weekend.

'I often trained alone and it was a test of my mental strength to go out in the cold and dark. I was also tired from looking after the kids. But I had my goal and it kept me going.

'I looked after the children all day and then went out training as soon as my husband walked through the door'

Unfortunately, my youngest son became ill three times during my training, so I had big gaps when he was in hospital. One of these gaps was just before the first qualifying race in

June 2005. He got better, so I was still able to compete, but didn't make the top five. I was bitterly disappointed. I came across the finish line, slumped down under a tree and wept.

'However, I still had one more chance as I'd signed up for another qualifying race in July – my last chance as I knew couldn't keep up that level of training for another year. During the race, I felt really good and

'I came over the finishing line proudly waving a Union Jack above my head'

had high hopes that I'd be in the top eight to get onto the reserve list, but it was not to be. I came close but not close enough and was devastated.

'Thankfully, we'd booked a long holiday in August so I went away with my family and had a relaxing month to get over my disappointment. However, when we arrived home and checked our email, I had a message telling me that some of the age-group winners had dropped out and I was in! I couldn't believe it – my dream had come true. The Championships were being held in Honolulu that October, so I hurriedly booked flights for the family and got back into training.

'I enjoyed it more than ever because I had no pressure. I knew I wasn't going to win, so my goal was not to be last in my age group (30–34). I ordered my much-coveted GB kit and bought pretty much everything – the tri suit, fleece, tracksuit, bag, cap – you name it, I bought it! When it arrived in the post,

I put the whole lot on and paraded around the house in it.

'We flew out a few days before the race and, when the big day came, I felt totally relaxed. It started at 7am on a very hot day and turned out to be a tough race with the heat and a strong headwind on the bike. But I didn't care about any of that – I loved it from start to finish and the whole experience was magic. Someone handed me a Union Jack on the finishing straight, so I came over the line proudly waving it above my head, with my family cheering madly from the sidelines. And I achieved my goal of not being last in my age group!

'My family were so proud. I think my husband was relieved that I'd achieved my goal – for a start, it meant he could see me in the evenings! I couldn't have done it without him.

'Two months later, I fell pregnant again, and had a third son, Arthur, in 2006. Three young boys is a lot to handle, so I've now got into cycle racing as the training is easier to fit in to my week. Triathlon will always hold a special place in my heart, though, and who knows what will happen when the kids are bit older and I have time to myself again! **99**

Carole's top training tip
'Enjoy your training – it's supposed to be fun! There were plenty of times I forgot this and it's good to remind yourself now and again.'

'TRIATHLON HAS TRANSFORMED MY LIFE'

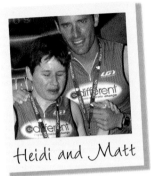

Heidi and Matt

Heidi Musser, 40, from Chicago, US, is the world's first blind female triathlete and has competed in about 30 triathlons, including two Escape From Alcatraz races.

66 I have been totally blind since birth. Sadly, this meant enduring a lot of prejudice and social isolation as a child, because teachers thought I was incapable of doing anything. During my early school years, I wasn't allowed to participate in assemblies or go on field trips and in my first year of high school I was made to listen to someone read about health and fitness during PE classes. My mother ended up teaching me Braille at home.

Years of feeling socially isolated fuelled an anger in me that eventually built up into wanting to show teachers, who doubted my potential, that I was capable of doing whatever I wanted.

'This started with a determination to go to university, and I gained a Bachelor of Arts degree in 1996. I then decided to start competing in sports events. I've been able to swim since I was small because my family took me to swim classes at our local YMCA. In August 1997, I became the first blind swimmer to participate in the Chicago Park District 2-Mile Swim in Lake Michigan. I swam with a guide next to me and was thrilled to be swimming alongside sighted competitors.

'After this triumph, I thought I could do anything. My YMCA coach suggested that I start training for

'I received a gold medal as the first blind female triathlete in the world'

triathlon. He taught me how to run on a treadmill and I could already cycle on a tandem bike. Two years later, I competed in the ITU Triathlon World Championships in Montreal, Canada, with a guide by my side (and as pilot on the tandem) and I received a gold medal as the first blind female triathlete in the world. When I returned home, people seemed to treat me with a new respect and I was invited to work as a Braille tutor in a local school.

'My triathlon career really took off when I was contacted by a man named

Matt Miller, who used to be an elite triathlete. He had heard about me through the Challenged Athletes Foundation (CAF) and wanted to be my guide. Even though I lived in Chicago and he in California, we did our first race together in 2001 (the Nautica Malibu triathlon). To swim in the Pacific Ocean was a new experience for me – I'm very light, so Matt had to grip his hands around my waist from

'We started at 7am and finished at 11.52pm, 9 minutes before the cut-off time'

the back and lift me over some of the more powerful waves. I have always been a fearless swimmer, though, and loved the whole experience.

'We turned out to be a great team – during a race Matt swims either next to me or behind me and I listen to his direction commands. For the bike section, we have a Griffen tandem specifically built for us. Matt rides in front as the pilot and I ride in the back as the stoker. During the run, we hold hands or sometimes use a flexible tether. If I'm feeling confident, I just run next to him, which enables me to swing both arms.

'Matt has changed my life. He respects and believes in me, and I've now participated in about 30 triathlons, including two Escape From Alcatraz races, which start at the famous island off the coast of San Francisco. It involves jumping off a ferry boat into freezing water and then swimming 1.5 miles in strong currents, riding a challenging 18-mile

bike course, followed by an 8-mile run through craggy trails. They were tough, but Matt was by my side to help me to the finish.

'In 2004, Matt had the bright idea that we should do an Ironman. I knew it would be an enormous challenge, but I decided to go for it. Matt put me in touch with four guides in the Chicago area and I trained with them for a year. On June 25, 2005, I competed in Ironman Coeur d'Alene, Idaho. We started at 7am. During the 2.4-mile swim, I swallowed quite a lot of water, but it otherwise went well. We had a fast bike leg, but I found the run really tough. We finished at 11:51pm with 9 minutes to spare before the cut-off time at midnight. I now hold the title of the world's first blind female Ironman (Ironwoman)!

'At school I had hardly any friends but now I have many. Triathlon has transformed my life and now other blind people have become athletes, too. Inspired by racing with me, Matt set up the C-Different Foundation (www.cdifferent.org), which matches up guides with blind or partially sighted athletes. I now participate in triathlons all over the world – I do it to inspire others and prove to people that if I can do it, they can do it too.'

Heidi's top training tip
'Don't over train! For me, triathlon is all about having fun and making friends.'

'TRIATHLON GAVE ME MY HEALTH BACK'

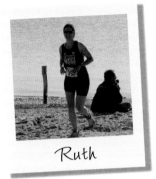

Ruth

Ruth Adams, 41, from Kentucky, US, recovered from gruelling cancer treatment with the help of triathlon…

❝In November 2002, I went to my doctor because I had a chest infection. She listened to my chest and suspected pneumonia, so requested an x-ray. This showed a shadow in my chest and I was sent for a biopsy. I was convinced I had lung cancer, but two agonising weeks later, my doctor confirmed that I had Hodgkin's lymphoma, a cancer of the lymphatic system. I was immediately referred to an oncologist to discuss treatment and saw it as the beginning of a journey that I was going to survive.

'In December 2002, I started chemotherapy to kill the tumour in my chest. Every other Friday for 6 months, I would spend the whole day having four different chemo drugs pumped into my body. It made me feel extremely ill and I would spend the fortnight in between trying to recover. I carried on teaching 2 days a week (I'm a professor of photography) as it was an important distraction and I did

lots of meditation to cope with the pain and nausea. I also took a photograph of myself every day to chronicle my treatment and recovery, and show others that you can survive.

'I saw it as the beginning of a journey that I was going to survive. I was adamant that I was not going to die'

'Chemo can affect your muscle mass and mine disappeared rapidly. I lost over 2 stone and slowly lost my hair, too. I tried to go for a short walk with my family every weekend to preserve at least some of my muscle mass and ate as healthily as I could.

'In May 2003, my chemo finished and I was given a month off to recover before starting radiation treatment to make sure every last cancer cell had been killed. I had 20 days of radiation. When treatment finally ended, there were no signs of active cancer cells, but my body was totally decimated. I couldn't walk for longer than

15 minutes and had no strength. To try and regain muscle, I spent the next few months going to gentle conditioning classes and taking short walks, but I had a long way to go before regaining the body I had before the cancer.

'My body was still so weak that 3 minutes of running felt like a lifetime!'

'In July 2004 my cousin told me he was doing a triathlon and we should all come and watch. I had assumed that all the participants would be über-athletes, but as I looked around, I realised that, apart from the people who were winning, everyone looked normal! I knew that I needed something to give me my health back, a goal to strive for, so my cousin's wife, my sister, my brother-in-law and I made a pact that we would do the race the following year.

'I had done no sport since school, so started off by following a really gentle running programme. My body was still so weak that 3 minutes of running felt like a lifetime. I also started swimming at the uni pool and met a woman there who told me about The Leukemia & Lymphoma Society's Team In Training, a programme that provides you with a trainer in return for raising money for the charity, so I got involved with them. I spent a year slowly but surely building my body up in preparation for the Long Island triathlon (a Super-Sprint). It was a struggle at times, but I desperately wanted my health back.

'When race day finally came, I was so nervous! But I had a ball – I was pleasantly surprised by how friendly everyone was on the course, with competitors cheering each other on. My whole family were there and my cousin and brother-in-law ran it with me – it was an incredible experience. I came over the line with my arms in the air and with my family cheering me on! Everybody was crying with happiness – here I was, recently out of cancer treatment, a month from my 40th birthday, completing my first triathlon.

'Triathlon empowered me and enabled me to get my health back – I've since done 7 sprint-distance and 3 Olympic-distance triathlons. My first Olympic-distance was as part of the Team In Training team – I raised almost $10,000 and raise more with each race I do.

I hope that I'm still doing triathlons well into the future – they are by far the greatest way to stay in shape without putting too much stress on one part of your body.

'I have to wait for five years after finishing treatment to be given the all-clear from the cancer – that will be July 2008 and the celebrations are going to be big! 99

Ruth's top training tip
'Remember, only a small per cent of the population take the time to even attempt to train for a triathlon, so be proud of yourself!'

199

'I RELY ON THE SURGE OF PEOPLE TO KNOW THAT WE'RE OFF!'

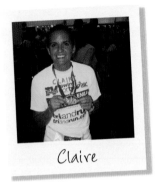

Claire

Claire Snell, 31, from London, has never let her deafness get in the way of a good challenge!

66 I've been deaf since birth and have 75% hearing loss – I can only hear loud bangs without my hearing aids. With my hearing aids, I can hear a lot more, but still rely on lip-reading. It's never stopped me doing sport, but has occasionally given me a few embarrassing moments – like the time I was waiting to do a floor routine in gymnastics but couldn't hear the music, so they announced over the tannoy that I needed silence to hear the music. The entire auditorium went silent and turned to watch me. Mortifying!

'As I got older, I became a gym-goer to stay in shape. I discovered triathlon when I was moaning to my friend Simon about how bored I was with my fitness regime. I'd never even heard of triathlon, but Simon persuaded me to sign up for a race with him.

My biggest challenge turned out to be the running. The feeling of my lungs hurting, the cold for the first few minutes, then being sweaty and hot – awful! I couldn't run for more

than 15 minutes without needing to stop and gasp for air. But I gradually learned to love it – I ran with a friend and we would natter and, later, I would run alone with some great tunes on my iPod, and make sure I ran somewhere where I could appreciate nature.

'I enjoyed the swim training, but couldn't hear the coach's instructions from the side of the pool – I had to ask people in the pool with me to

'I couldn't run for more than 15 minutes without needing to stop and gasp for air'

repeat the instructions, so I could lipread. By the time race day came around, I was terrified! I hadn't done nearly enough bike training, and all my running had been on the flat, so my stomach did a flip when I arrived to discover that there were two HUGE hills in the running section! I really hadn't a clue what I was meant to be doing and was late getting to the poolside, so was frantically pulling on my swim cap even as I was getting into the water! Once I got started, it

'Cycling was always my weakest discipline (I sometimes go so slowly up hills, I'm on the verge of wobbling over)'

was a bit mad in the pool – I was slowed down a bit by other people, got kicked a few times, and ended up just giggling at the ridiculousness of it all!

'My cycling was always my weakest discipline (I sometimes go so slowly up hills, I'm on the verge of wobbling over), so I decided to just enjoy the country route, which was really scenic. That weird bit of running after cycling really does happen – it feels like running through jelly! I really had done no hill running and my poor legs didn't know what hit them when the hills loomed up, but I got lots of extra cheering from the runners alongside me, which really helped. I have to confess that I bawled as I ran under the finish clock and into my boyfriend's arms!

'Two years later, I decided to brave an Olympic-distance with an open-water swim. I trained more intensively this time, but when the day of the race came round, I still felt really daunted by the swim – my breathing gets panicky when I get into cold water, and I had to tell myself to breathe calmly when I got in. I couldn't hear the starter gun, so just relied on the

surge of people to let me know we were off! It was a cold swim, but once I was out of the water, I looked back thinking, "that's brilliant, I've done it, now I can have fun" – and I did! The rest of the race was fantastic.

'Doing a few races made me realise that I really rely on having friends with me at the beginning – I can't swim with my hearing aids in, so I need my friends to repeat any instructions that are issued by the marshals. I've been lucky enough to have my friend Emma at my last three tris, and Simon and my friend Jen at my first one. And my transitions are never going to be

'Hearing aids are a fiddle to get in when you're shaking from excitement'

speedy because I wear my hearing aids for the bike and run and they are a fiddle to get in when you're shaking from excitement!

'My goal now is to do an Olympic-distance in under 2½ hours. Tri is definitely the sport for me – it's made my muscles super-sleek and, best of all, there's the huge buzz you get when you cross the finish line knowing you've completed a demanding race that few people dare to do! 99

Claire's top training tip
'Imagine the crowds cheering you across the finish line – I visualise it whenever I'm feeling low during training!'

'IT'S MY ESCAPE, MY TIME TO SWITCH OFF'

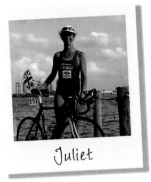

Juliet

Juliet Vickery, 44, from Cambridge, immersed herself in triathlon training to help her cope with grief.

66 I took up triathlon ten years ago when I first moved to Cambridge. I'd moved down from Scotland, where I used to do hill running, and wanted to do something new, so I joined Cambridge Triathlon Club. I'd also been injured a few times as a result of my running, so thought the cross-training might do me some good.

'Over the next few years, I developed a real passion for the sport and, with the help of other club members, I started coming in the top three of my age group in races. In 1999, my husband David and I had our daughter, Freya. The pregnancy was a breeze and I was able to take up training again soon afterwards – I even raced in the World Championships in 2000! In 2002, we decided to try for a second child and I fell pregnant quite quickly. This pregnancy was also a breeze, until September 2003. Four days before the baby was due, I realised that I hadn't felt it move for a while. At this stage

of pregnancy, it can move a lot and you really feel it, so I knew something was wrong. I went for a scan, which showed that there was no longer a heartbeat and my baby had died in the womb. I can't really describe how I felt. I was in pieces – it was the worst experience of my life and the next few weeks were a blur of grief.

'Within weeks, I felt strongly that I needed an escape and a distraction

'I was in pieces – it was the worst experience of my life and the next few weeks were a blur of grief'

from my grief, which was threatening to overwhelm me. I knew that I wanted to try for another baby, but I didn't want to start until I had got my body strong and fit again, as I hadn't really trained much during the pregnancy.

'I set myself the goal of the Duathlon World Championships the following year – I chose duathlon (run, bike, run) because it was earlier in the year than the Triathlon World Championships and I wanted to wait only six months before trying for another baby. I immersed myself in the training and found that it was incredibly cathartic. It was my time to switch off from thinking about my lost baby – when I ran, I thought about my breathing and my pace; when I swam, I emptied my mind by thinking about my stroke. Cycling was the only discipline where sometimes I would

'I would often find myself crying when I went out alone on long bike rides in the country'

think about the baby – I would often find myself crying when I went out alone on long bike rides in the country.

'The people at my triathlon club were incredibly supportive – they knew why I was doing it and helped in any way they could.

'The training paid off and, six months later, I took silver at the Championships. At the procession afterwards, a female triathlete I had met at previous races came up to me and said, "I know why you're here", and then burst into tears and gave me a big hug of support. I experienced this kind of thing so many times from people in the triathlon community and it really meant a lot.

'Although I was still grieving, I felt ready to try for another baby and fell pregnant again within weeks, but sadly it was to be the first of five miscarriages over the next three years. The doctors don't know the cause, but each time I lost a baby, it had

common chromosomal problems that nothing could be done about.

'After each loss, I would throw myself back into training to help me cope. Last year, I qualified to compete for Great Britain, but had to drop out of the race because I fell pregnant. But I miscarried again and found that time especially hard to cope with as I knew it could well be the last chance for another child. Having missed out on the GB race, I decided that I would aim to get a national ranking by coming in the top three at a race in Wales two months later. I achieved my goal at the race and am now ranked second in the country for my age group.

At times, triathlon may have been too much of an escape – it doesn't take the pain away, but ultimately it has carried me through times that I would struggle to have survived if I hadn't had an outlet. It restored some of my self-confidence and helped me feel in control of my body when I felt it was letting me down so badly in other ways.

'Whatever life throws at me next I know that triathlon and triathletes will be there with me. It will always be part of my life and I plan to still be competing on my zimmer frame! 99

Juliet's top training tip
'Always have your swim and run kit with you – you never know when you might be able to fit in a session.'

Go clubbing

Joining a triathlon club may seem like an intimidating thing to do, but in fact it's just the opposite! Most clubs (depending on their size) cater for everyone from total beginners to elite triathletes. Here are some of the reasons you might consider joining one, now or in the future.

You get great advice

'The diversity of athletes in triathlon clubs mean you will benefit from the wisdom of more seasoned triathletes, as well as people who can remember what it's like to be a beginner,' says elite triathlete Olly Freeman. From how to train and what to eat, to which races are best and what bike to buy, other members and the club's coaches will be great sources of advice.

It improves your training

As part of your membership fee, triathlon clubs have weekly coached sessions in each of the disciplines. If you're a beginner, this will help you to learn the ropes and increase your confidence. If you've done a few triathlons and want to improve, coached sessions will really bring on both your technique and fitness levels. Having fixed sessions to attend can boost your motivation: 'You're likely to find a training buddy who's a similar level or just a bit better than you to keep you on your toes and give your training a bit of a competitive edge,' says Freeman.

It's sociable

Triathlon clubs are a great place to meet new people with similar interests to you. They usually organise plenty of social events, you will have companions to go to races with (and give you a lift!) and you don't have to train alone. 'It's really nice to see a friendly face when you turn up for an early-morning swim!' says Freeman. Having company is also handy during the dark evenings of winter when it's safer to train with other people.

You get to wear cool kit!

Most triathlon clubs have their own kit emblazoned with the name of the club, which you can buy to race in. It makes you look and feel like a professional, even if you aren't!

How to find a club

The British Triathlon Federation is the governing body and its website has a list of every club in the country. Visit www.britishtriathlon.org. Each club's contact details are on there, so give them a call or send an email with any questions you have and tell them what level of triathlete you are. You can usually go along for a session to see if you like it before deciding whether or not to join.

Further information

Log on to...

... one of the following inspiring triathlon websites – they are packed with useful training tips:

www.beginnertriathlete.com

An US site with a friendly forum as well as some excellent training plans and beginner-specific tips.

www.tri247.com

A well-designed UK site packed with expert information and training plans, and a section on women-only events and training camps.

www.britishtriathlon.org

The home page of the British Triathlon Federation, this is a useful resource for race and club information. If you are planning on doing a number of triathlons, it is recommended you join the BTF, as you will get reduced entry fees to a variety of races.

Further reading

If you want to focus on a particular aspect of your training, pick up a book.

Running Made Easy

by Susie Whalley and Lisa Jackson (Collins & Brown, £9.99)
The predecessor to *Triathlon Made Easy*, written by *Zest* writers, this is an inspiring beginner's guide to running.

Master The Art of Swimming

by Steven Shaw
(Collins & Brown, £12.99)
Takes you through each step of the stroke cycle for breaststroke, crawl, backstroke and butterfly.

7-week Cycling for Fitness

by Chris Sidwells (DK, £9.99)
A great beginner's guide to biking with step-by-step advice on technique.

Zest magazine

The UK's bestselling health and fitness glossy. To subscribe, log on to www.zest.co.uk

Book into...

... a residential triathlon camp designed for beginners and improvers.

Tri Camp UK

Run by triathlon trainer John Sullivan, who created our core and body conditioning programme, Tri Camp UK offers affordable weekend training camps across the UK with swim, bike and run coaches for all abilities.
www.tricampuk.com

adidas Eyewear Triathlon Training Camp

If you fancy something a little sunnier, professional triathlete and trainer Richard Allen runs regular training camps in Greece in association with adidas and Neilson holidays.
www.neilson.co.uk/beachplus/triathlon

Contact us

If this book has inspired you to take up triathlon training, or helped you improve your performance, we would love to hear from you. Email us at zoe.mcdonald@natmags.co.uk or lisa.buckingham@yahoo.co.uk and let us know how you get on!

Index

A huge thank you to…

Alison Pylkkänen and the *Zest* team, for their ideas and support, particularly *Zest*'s resident Ironwoman, Andrea Sullivan.

Zest's art director Kelly Flood, stylists Marianne De Vries and Kelly Moseley, and picture editor Caroline Willingham for their vision and style in helping to create the fantastic photographs and cover of this book, and to photographers Derek Lomas and Neil Cooper. Thank you also to Libby Willis, our eagle-eyed proofreader, Abby Franklin, our designer and Miriam Hyslop, our patient editor.

The inspiring bank of experts, trainers and athletes who supported us throughout the research and writing process. Thanks go in particular to Bill Black for his time, good humour and willingness to help us with the training plans. Likewise Helen Gorman of Zoggs, Malcolm Balk, Steven Shaw, Martin Yelling, John Sullivan of TriCampUK.com, Laura Denham-Jones, Purple Patch Running, Ralph Hydes, Graham Walton (www.wilsoncycles.co.uk), Scott Bentley, Two Wheels Good bike shop, London (www.twowheelsgood.co.uk) and everyone at SBI PR, which represents the Michelob Ultra London Triathlon, particularly Jo Taylor.

The brands who helped us with our kit sections and put us in touch with experts – Zoggs, Trek Bikes, Tri Girl (www.trigirl.co.uk), SBR, Aqua Sphere, Asics, Nike, Speedo, sweatyBetty, Weightloss Resources and WeightWatchers.

To the incredible case studies for their participation, and to the organisations and charities that helped us find them.

Zoë's thanks
An enormous thank you to Tarquin, my husband, an incredible support throughout the writing process, and to my family. Thank you too, to all the friends and colleagues who offered their encouragement and input.

Lisa's thanks
Huge thanks to my boyfriend Tim for providing endless lovely dinners, back rubs and support during the writing process. I couldn't have done it without you. And to all my friends for their encouragement and patiently listening to me talk endlessly about triathlon!